GMOs:
What's Hidden In Our Food

How It Affects Our Health,
The Environment & Politics
In America

PART 1 of a 3 Part Series

Michele Jacobson

ISBN: 978-0692256343

NUTRITION PRESCRIPTION LLC
www.nutritionprescription.biz

"GMO crops were planted on about 169 million acres in the U.S. in 2013, about half the total land used for crops." (*USDA*)

———————————

Genetically engineered foods have infiltrated the
American food supply,
and despite grassroots efforts to
enforce mandatory labeling
they largely remain invisible to the general public.

Education on this issue is key!

Learn how GMOs impact your health,
the environment and politics.

Once you know the facts,
you won't be able to close your eyes.

TABLE OF CONTENTS - PART I

INTRODUCTION

Presumptuous as it may sound, I think everyone should read this book. Everyone who eats food, who cares about the environment, who cares about wildlife or about their political rights. If you fall into any of these categories you deserve to be informed on the topic of GMOs.

It's written so that it can be easily understood by young and old alike, and everyone in-between. It does not include information that is undocumented or sensationalistic. This book will tell you what you need to know about GMOs and how they affect *you*.

If you shop and cook for your family, you'll want to know the information that is in this book. If you simply *eat*, you'll want to know it, too. Some of the information may be familiar to you, as the acronym GMO has become a familiar one in the United States over the past few years. Read on, and you will garner so much more than the mere snippets the media puts out there for the general public.

GMOs have not only pervaded the vast majority of the foods we eat; they have also negatively impacted wildlife and the environment, affected the reproduction of plant-life, and compromised the very fabric of our political system since their inception. Without mandatory GMO labeling in place, the American public has been deprived of knowing what the majority of their food contains, at its basest level. Indeed, were it not for the citizens of the United States themselves, and their grassroots efforts, chances are we'd be unaware of the acronym GMO at all.

CHAPTER 1

WHAT ARE GMOs?

GMO stands for Genetically Modified Organism. You may sometimes see the initials GE, which stands for genetically engineered, or the word transgenic, which is synonymous as well. According to the World Health Organization, GMOs occur when the genetic material in an organism "has been altered in a way that does not occur naturally." Period.

Although this may be the official definition, it only tells part of the story. Genetic modification, or engineering, is the *unnatural* alteration of the DNA of a seed in a laboratory. It occurs when the genes from the DNA of one species is extracted and *artificially* forced into the genes of an unrelated plant or animal. The foreign genes can come from bacteria, viruses, insects, animals, or even humans. It never occurs in nature, the procedure is always executed in a laboratory.

People sometimes question what the difference is between genetic engineering and *selective breeding*, in which an animal is bred, or a plant is grafted, in an effort to bring forth particular traits. The difference is that selective breeding can occur in nature and the genuses are the same. For example: a cockapoo is a mixture of a cocker spaniel and a poodle; it's mammals and mammals. This particular type of cross-breeding is one most of us are familiar with; perhaps it is done to produce a pet that is hypo-allergenic, or doesn't shed, or that is smaller in size. Another good example is the common grapefruit, which is actually a *hybrid* of a pummelo and a sweet orange. A hybrid is the offspring of two plants of different breeds. The grapefruit was developed by farmers, but there are other hybrid fruits of unknown origin, such as boysenberries, which have evolved by themselves over time. No scientists, no geneticists, no laboratories. Because hybrids are simply cross-breeds between the same genuses they can occur by themselves in nature. Proponents of GMOs often liken the process of genetic engineering to hybridization or cross-breeding by saying that what they are doing is "nothing new," but with the above simple examples we can see this isn't the case.

Genetic engineering is generally done to bring forth some desirable (desirable to *whom* can be questionable) trait in a seed or plant. Let's go back to the first genetically engineered plant, the Flavr Savr tomato, which was brought to market in the early 1990's. According to the biotech company Calgene, it was "genetically altered to ripen longer on the vine while remaining firm for picking and shipping, characteristics that should make it more flavorful and last longer than most other tomatoes on the market." In other words, it was genetically engineered not to start its decline in freshness shortly after being picked, as ripe tomatoes are prone to do. Extending freshness, reducing spoilage; it seemed like they had a good idea. Interestingly, Calgene *willingly* put stickers on the Flavr Savr tomatoes, as well as brochures at the point of sale in supermarkets, so that consumers would have a better understanding of the genetic engineering process. The tomato - touted as a gourmet product and sold at a premium price - was sold from 1994 to 1997, but was then pulled from the market. There are conflicting reports of why the project didn't succeed; either Calgene didn't handle the marketing well, the tomatoes - though ripe and red - were too soft, or if there was a lack of consumer demand due to the genetic modification process.1 After the tomato was pulled, Calgene sold the rights to the biotech company, Monsanto.

Public outrage against GMOs isn't anything new, because even in the 1970's the Flavr Savr was immediately condemned by critics of genetic engineering. The F.D.A was also ridiculed for claiming the tomato was nutritionally identical to conventional tomatoes. Said Jeremy Rifkin of the Pure Food Campaign at the time, "Consumers have a right to know if there is something different in their food..." Sound familiar?

Whether you agree with the ethics of genetic engineering or not, what may have started out with good intentions, to actually improve the durability of a fresh product, has now turned infinitely more sinister.

Today, for the most part, seeds are genetically engineered to either produce their own pesticides in an effort to ward off insects, or to resist the effects of herbicides, such as glyphosate. This is the active ingredient in Roundup, a weed-killer which is generally mass-sprayed over crops and farms. If a seed has been genetically engineered to be resistant to the effects of glyphosate, then the spraying can be done en-mass and the plant itself won't die. If the seed is genetically engineered to act as a pesticide, it means that every single cell of the plant will contain this pesticide in its DNA.

The American public is expected to eat these plants as their food. To reiterate, not only are the seeds genetically engineered to *contain* the herbicides and insecticides as part of their DNA, they are also then being topically *sprayed* with toxins. *This is our food.*

So here we are, roughly 20 years after the Flavr Savr tomato, and an alarming 85 - 95% of the following crops planted in the United States today are genetically engineered: *corn, soybeans, sugar beets, canola* and *cotton.* These are known as the big five. You may be thinking to yourself "Well, I don't eat beets" or "I'm not a vegetarian, so I don't eat soy products." However, the following information may surprise you.

Corn and Maize

Maize, or corn, is genetically engineered to resist both insects and weeds. Since 1997, the year that it first started to be grown in the U.S., the percentage of this crop that is genetically modified has skyrocketed to a staggering 88%. The maize is also grown in numerous countries around the world, most notably in India. There are many different varieties of GMO maize, but the two most prevalent are Roundup maize (which is resistant to weeds) and Bt corn (which is genetically engineered with the insecticide built in). Though the majority of maize grown worldwide is used for animal feed, this still presents problems for humans who want to avoid GMOs in the food they eat (this is covered more fully in Alfalfa, below). The more pressing problems emanate from foods that are produced directly from genetically engineered crops.

Do you eat breakfast cereal? Cornflakes are made from "cored maize which has been milled to maize grits or flakes."[2] If you aren't purchasing organic cereal, you have no way of knowing if you're eating GMOs. However, since 88% of the American maize crop is planted with genetically modified seed, well...you can do the math.

Do you use corn oil, or a product labeled 'vegetable oil' that may have a high percentage of corn oil as an ingredient? Chances are overwhelming that it's a GMO product.

Do you simply *eat* corn? Corn on the cob, canned corn, frozen corn or any food containing corn (vegetable soup, for example)? In 2011, the biotech company Monsanto (you'll be hearing that name quite a bit in this book) began to plant its genetically modified sweet corn seed. This initial planting accounted for roughly 40% of the sweet corn market in the United States.[3] Largely unbeknownst to consumers, the corn began to be sold just in time for the summer season of 2012, not only in the supermarket, but at farmers' markets and farm stands across the country. It might *look* like farm-fresh corn, and it is...just from a farm where GMO seed is sown and genetically engineered corn is grown.

Do you ever eat processed foods, like cookies, cakes or ice cream? Read the label: if it's not an organic product, and if it contains corn starch (modified food starch), corn flour, corn syrup or high fructose corn syrup (HFCS), you can almost assume that it was made with genetically engineered corn.

Though it is possible to purchase organic corn syrup, this is not the case for high fructose corn syrup. HFCS is a highly processed product and, as such, contains chemicals that render it non-organic. This substance has been linked to the scourges of obesity and type 2 diabetes that plague our society.[4] Shockingly, according to the USDA website outlining the myriad usages for corn, "(g)overnment programs have been instrumental in the development of...HFCS."[5] All for the expansion of the American corn market.

However, here's something good to chew on: popcorn is *not* a GMO crop (though I still recommend you buy organic)!

Soybeans

So you're not a vegetarian? You can bet that soybeans or their derivatives still most assuredly find their way into your diet. Primarily used as food additives and animal feed, soy is the crop most likely to be genetically modified: 94% of seeds planted in the United States in 2011 were GMO. "Soybeans currently surpass both corn and cotton as the genetically engineered crop with the greatest planted acreage."[6] So, statistically, whatever way you want to slice it, soy is the one to watch out for. For vegetarians, this issue could very well be an easier one to spot, as the less-processed soy foods such as tofu and tempe, for example, are the ones that are more likely to be produced and labeled either as "Non-GMO" or 'organic', a certification that ensures a product is GMO-free. However, of the approximately 3.06 billion bushels of soybeans planted in the U.S. - we are the largest producer and exporter of soy in the world - 70 million bushels are genetically modified for resistance to the herbicide, glyphosate.[7] Once again, this genetic modification not only provides the plants with the herbicide as part of their DNA, after planting they are then *sprayed* with the herbicide so that the encroaching weeds are killed but the the plants themselves survive. Dinner is served.

When soybeans are not eaten in their whole state (i.e. edamame), or in more recognizable formulations (i.e. tofu, tempe or soy milk), they are utilized for an overwhelming supply of products and additives in our food system. In addition to traditional soy products such as miso and soy sauce, which are produced from whole soy beans, there is soybean oil, soy flour, infant soy formula, soy meat substitutes and extenders, soy dairy substitutes and extenders, "fake" products (which are highly processed), and additives that hide in processed foods. An example of this is soy lecithin, which acts as an emulsifier that stabilizes products such as ice cream, margarine and baked goods. In addition, a large portion of processed soy, in the form of soymeal and husks, is used as animal feed.

There has been public outrage concerning the ongoing usage of GMOs in baby formula. Present in soy milk, as well as other ingredients found in formula, such as rBGH dairy, corn syrup, and sugar from sugar beets (all discussed below), the GMO products were enough to play havoc with the emotions of parents wanting the best for their babies. As a result of this the premium organic segment of the baby food market has grown "at an average annual rate of 43% from 2010 to 2012."[8] Despite the uproar about baby formula and its questionable ingredients, brand names Gerber, Similac and Enfamil - which combined account for more than 90% of all formula sold in the U.S. - have refused to obliterate GMOs from their conventional products.

Since 1997, the soybean has only been genetically engineered to resist insects and weeds, but in November, 2013, biotech companies Monsanto and DuPont Pioneer broke the news that they had a new plan for modifying the humble legume. Capitalizing on the FDA's intent to reduce trans-fats in foods,[9] they announced a genetically engineered soybean with a new and altered composition of fats. Take note, this is *not* the soybean nature created. Said the Director of Food and Industry Markets at biotech company DuPont Pioneer, about the new genetically engineered soybean: "(i)t almost mirrors olive oil in terms of the composition of fatty acids...In essence we've rebuilt the profile."[10] So, is this truly still a *soybean*? An oil produced from these new soybeans is already available to restaurants and food companies in limited quantities; yep, you already might be eating it. The biotech companies are betting the consumer embraces this genetically engineered product because it provides a benefit to *them*: the health benefit of decreased trans-fats. They are also hoping restaurants want it because the new oil stays fresher, for longer periods of time. This will enable establishments to change their frying oil less frequently. *But wait!* As a consumer, you *want* a restaurant to change their frying oil frequently - every day, in fact - otherwise free radicals build up in the old, used oil and can quickly become carcinogenic.[11] So, who is *really* benefitting here? The biotech company that sells the seeds for the genetically altered soybeans? The restaurants that use less oil? Surely not the consumer.

So, if someone questions your organic edamame, point out that it isn't the innocent soybean to beware of; it's the genetically engineered, processed soy products that lurk in almost every packaged and processed food that is the demon. As usual, the devil is in the details.

Sugar Beets

If you think white crystals of sugar are processed only from stalks of sugarcane, think again. While it's true that sugarcane once provided the world's only source of sugar, today about 45% of the stuff is now processed from sugar beets. The two crops don't compete for the same land; sugar cane grows in warm climates and sugar beets only grow in cooler climates. Russia is the top producer nation of sugar beets in the world. While sugar cane is not a genetically engineered crop, sugar beets most assuredly are. In 2008 - the first year they were cultivated in the U.S., half the total crop was genetically engineered. Today, fully 95% of sugar beets grown in the U.S. are genetically engineered to withstand the spraying of glyphosate (Monsanto's herbicide, Roundup).

Interestingly, though sugar from GMO sugar beets has been approved for both human consumption and animal feed in numerous countries; to date, commercial *production* and *planting* has only been approved in the U.S. and Canada. Twenty percent of our domestic sugar comes from sugar beets - again, 95% GMO - with the remaining pulp used for animal feed.

According to the Sugar Industry Biotech Council "...sugar is the same no matter its original plant source or growing practice. Sugar – whether from sugar beets or sugar cane, or from sugar crops grown using conventional, biotech, or organic methods – is pure and natural and has the same nutritional value, composition and wholesomeness."[12] Their list of processed food and beverage products that may include sugar derived from biotech crops includes the following: candy bars, cakes, cookies, pies, bread, bagels, donuts, muffins, sweet rolls, snack crackers, chips, ice cream, sherbet, yogurt, breakfast cereals, toaster pastries, waffles, fruit drinks and juices, soft drinks, salad dressings, ketchup, barbecue sauce, jams, jellies, whipped toppings and confections.

The information distributed by the Sugar Industry Biotech Council seems discomforting since, compared with other crops, genetically engineered sugar beets require the most intensive and frequent use of weed control products.[13] What this means, and please excuse the redundancy, is that the sugar beet is genetically engineered at the molecular level to resist the effects of the herbicide glyphosate. Then, as it grows it is sprayed - *intensively* and *frequently* - with this herbicide, a known toxin.

A spoonful of GMOs in your morning coffee? I think not. Organic cane sugar - GMO-free - is readily available.

Canola

Although some people think they are the same, canola and rapeseed are different. Canola actually emanates from two words: 'can' comes from Canada, where it was invented, and 'ola' stands for oil. Canola was developed as a cultivar of rapeseed in the early 1970's using traditional plant breeding methods as to assure the plants' safety for human and animal consumption, and it differs from the non-edible rapeseed only slightly.[14] Today, it is an important crop, not just for cooking oil and margarine, but because the raw material is also used for animal feed and industrial purposes, many of them eco-friendly.

Approximately 90% of the U.S. canola crop is genetically engineered to be herbicide resistant. By now you know what that means.

Canola oil is touted as a healthy oil due to its high levels of monounsaturated fats, as well as its low levels of saturated fats. Indeed, the U.S. Food and Drug Administration provides the qualified health claim that: "Limited and not conclusive scientific evidence suggests that eating about one and a half tablespoons (19 grams) of canola oil daily may reduce the risk of coronary heart disease due to the unsaturated fat content in canola oil. To achieve this possible benefit, canola oil is to replace a similar amount of saturated fat and not increase the total number of calories you eat in a day."[15]

Low levels of saturated fat also make canola oil attractive to food producers looking to reduce or eliminate saturated or trans fats in their foods. So is canola oil a healthy oil? Sure, but only if it's non-GMO canola oil.

Cotton

You might not think of cotton as a food product at all. As a matter of fact, you might be thinking you've noticed high-end clothing labels touting their product as made from organic cotton (and your subsequent shock at the price tag). Well, once you hear that cotton is considered the world's "dirtiest crop" you might think the price of organic cotton garb is worth it. "Eight of the top 10 pesticides most commonly used on U.S. conventionally produced cotton were classified as moderately to highly hazardous by the World Health Organization."[16] With 90% of the U.S. cotton crop genetically engineered to resist both insects and herbicides (some recent statistics put that figure as high as 98%), you can easily recognize why organic cotton duds would be sold at a premium price.

While it's true that cotton is primarily known as a textile, it is also used around the world for animal feed (cottonseed meal) and is very much present in our food supply as cottonseed oil. However it also lurks in many processed foods on the market today. Have you seen these words on the ingredient list of your favorite foods: cellulose (a thickening and binding agent made from a by-product of cotton), methylcellulose (a thickening agent), thickeners, stabilizers and/or emulsifiers? Present in products such as dressings, meats and sausages, baked goods, chewing gum, ice cream and fiber fortified diet products, to name a few, they are all a by-product of cotton.[17] And you thought cotton was just the clothes on your back.

As you can tell, GMO crops have wheedled their way into the vast majority of processed foods in the American marketplace. Seventy-five to eighty percent of the processed foods in your supermarket contain GMOs, and the American consumer is largely unaware. Why? There are two simple reasons:

1- They may not even know what GMOs are.

2- There is no mandatory GMO labeling in the United States.

GMOs can also hide in foods where you wouldn't expect to find them. Even when you think you're eating "healthy," it's possible you might be eating genetically engineered foods. The following fruits and vegetables are routinely genetically engineered: zucchini, yellow summer squash and Hawaiian "Rainbow" papaya. Genetically engineered ingredients can also hide in milk and dairy products that aren't labeled "organic" or "made without rBGH."

rBGH

rBGH stands for recombinant Bovine Growth Hormone; indeed, the very word *recombinant* means "formed by laboratory methods." rBGH is a genetically engineered hormone - a synthetic variation of a natural pituitary hormone - that is injected into dairy cows to increase their milk production. It was developed by the biotech company Monsanto, and recently sold to Elanco, a division of Eli Lily. Approved by the FDA in 1993, and in use since 1994, the major public backlash against rBGH began sometime around 2007 for a multitude of reasons. Americans, in general, do not like it when animals are mistreated, and when dairy cows are injected with artificial growth hormones, for the purpose of producing about a gallon more of milk per day, they are more susceptible to mastitis, an infection of the udders. This, in turn, means more antibiotics for the animal; a vicious cycle for the dairy cows and more antibiotics in the end food product. rBGH usage has also been linked to reproductive issues in the cows.[18] Though several early studies showed that milk with rBGH was higher in IFG-1 (insulin-like growth factor-1) and linked to an increased risk of breast, prostate, colorectal and other cancers, subsequent studies showed a weaker relationship. The American Cancer Society, however, encourages expanded research on this issue, and also on the effects of increased usage of antibiotics as a result of rBGH. However, according to the Cancer Prevention Coalition, "(a)s detailed in a January 1996 report in the prestigious International Journal of Health Services, rBGH milk differs from natural milk chemically, nutritionally, pharmacologically and immunologically, besides being contaminated with pus and antibiotics resulting from mastitis induced by the biotech hormone."[19] As a result of this information going public, the sale of organic milk, free of rBGH and rBST (another form of the hormone) grew in leaps and bounds. This, despite an odd and short-lived campaign of disclaimers on containers of *conventional* milk brands *using* rBGH, which claimed that the milk was just the same as organic milk. (A bizarre marketing twist.)

Although it is banned in the EU, Canada, New Zealand and Australia, at this writing 40% of the milk on the American market still contains the artificial hormone. That said, it's pretty easy to find conventional brands of milk that are rBGH-free, even if you don't buy organic (which by regulation cannot contain artificial hormones).

But what about all the other dairy products that you like to eat? The yogurt, ice cream, cheese, butter, cream cheese, cottage cheese, puddings, sour cream, even whipped cream? If these products are not labeled as containing milk from 'cows not treated with rBGH' - and some are prominently labeled - then you have no way of knowing if they do or do not contain the GE hormone! You might be very aware of the "No rBGH" advisory on the carton of milk you buy, but completely unmindful of it with the other dairy products in which milk is an ingredient.

The "Rainbow" Papaya

In a blessed agricultural climate, papaya is Hawaii's fifth largest crop, trailing after marijuana, pineapples, sugarcane, macadamia nuts and coffee.[20] Though papaya is not native to Hawaii, it thrived there. That is, until the Papaya ringworm virus got to it.

The Hawaiian "Rainbow" papaya - if you read the papaya by-lines - sounds like a fantastic success story. The only commercially grown genetically engineered fruit available in the United States, it accounts for approximately 80% of the 30 million pounds of papaya harvested in Hawaii annually. Here's a bit of history: between the 1950's and the 1990's, the Hawaiian papaya crop was plagued by the Papaya ringspot virus, also known as PRV. After the groves were hopscotched from island to island in an effort to thwart the disease - which is primarily spread by aphids - a scientist named Dr. Dennis Gonsalves developed a genetically engineered resistant strain of the fruit. Released in 1998, the transgenic "Rainbow" papaya is inoculated with a gene from the ringspot virus itself, basically giving it immunity to the virus. In effect, the papaya had a virus, so it was "vaccinated" by altering genes to produce a tiny piece of the virus in each cell. This triggered the papayas immune system.

Prior to the development of the "Rainbow" genetically engineered papaya, consuming fruit with the ringspot virus was not problematic as PRV does not infect humans; indeed, papaya with ringspot has been eaten by people for a very long time. Indeed, "(t)here are no impacts to human health from affected plants and fruit."[21] Most negatively affected is the farmer, as crop growth is stunted. Regardless, the "Rainbow" papaya has now been commercially grown in Hawaii since 1999, and is approved in both the United States and Canada, though not in the EU, where both its import and marketing are prohibited.

The transgenic "Rainbow" may have seemed like a godsend for the Hawaiian papaya industry, but it has hardly been a panacea. For one thing, it is *not* resistant to strains of PRV emanating from other countries that grow papaya, and "(e)xposure to foreign strains of the virus is a serious risk, as "Rainbow" papayas have been shown to be susceptible to PRSV from Guam, Taiwan and Thailand."[22] The GE plants have been known to contaminate - via air and seed - both the conventional and organic crops of papaya which still exist on Hawaii, though these crops are in the minority.[23] Sadly, "(l)ess than 15% of the papayas grown in the State of Hawaii can make the claim of being non-GMO."[24]

Export of the fruit is also a problem, as many countries reject any food that is genetically modified. (Japan, which constitutes 20% of Hawaii's export market for papaya, had initially been resistant to importing the GE fruit; however since 2011 they've approved the fruit for import.) Sales values have been down every year since the transgenic "Rainbow" fruit was introduced.[25]

Monsanto now owns the patent on the transgenic "Rainbow" papaya.

Alfalfa

In January, 2011, amidst stiff public opposition, the unrestricted nationwide planting of genetically engineered alfalfa was approved by the USDA. While you may not think this affects you, since alfalfa isn't something you would actually eat, read on.

As the fourth largest crop in America, alfalfa is a massive moneymaker for Monsanto and Forage Genetics (a subsidiary of Land O'Lakes), the two companies that developed the seed. The vehicle utilized for genetic modification was the E. coli bacteria. As a GM Roundup Ready seed, farmers can spray the toxic herbicide glyphosate freely without harming the crop. Although the alfalfa is grown primarily to make hay for animal feed; remember, what an animal eats can ultimately find its way into your stomach as well (if you eat the animal, of course).

A major problem with genetically engineered alfalfa is the high likelihood of contamination to conventional non-genetically engineered, as well as organic alfalfa fields. This is an especially huge issue for the organic meat industry. Organic meat can only be certified as such if the animals have consumed organic feed or, alternatively, are grass-fed or pastured. If said animals graze on grass which has been contaminated with GE alfalfa, or eat tainted alfalfa or hay, the meat can no longer be certified organic. The knowledge that GE alfalfa pollen is flying around and may contaminate his fields is enough to make any farmer - and especially an *organic* farmer - pick up and leave town. Organic farming is a costly and labor intensive process in itself, the prospect of discovering at harvest-time that your product cannot be certified is enough to make a farmer kick the bucket.

Organic meat isn't the only commodity at risk; organic dairy farmers also rely upon organic hay to feed their cows. If there is any risk of contamination to the organic alfalfa, then everybody bears the brunt. Organic alfalfa or hay becomes more difficult for dairy farmers to obtain, and ultimately makes organic dairy prices rise. Worse for the farmers, worse for the consumers who want to buy their organic dairy products.[26]

The USDA did not test the genetically engineered alfalfa for its effects on humans or animals prior to approving unrestricted planting in 2011. Fast forward to 2013 and reports of contamination began to surface, as was predicted. The USDA, to date, has refused to investigate the issue.

Summer Squash and Zucchini

These varieties of squash are routinely genetically engineered to eliminate the risk of a number of different viral diseases which they are particularly prone to. Genetically engineered yellow crookneck squash and its cousin, green zucchini, have been available since 1995. They are engineered to be resistant to the watermelon mosaic virus, zucchini yellow mosaic virus and cucumber mosaic virus. Of the approximately 45,000 acres of squash planted in in the U.S. in 2012, 25,000 acres were from genetically engineered seed, roughly over 50%.

However, humble squash have a tale to tell about mother nature's grand design. It seems that perhaps these viruses had a *purpose*, because there have been some unintended consequences since genetically engineered squash have been brought to the fields. Cucumber beetles are a natural pest of squash, and they seem to have a preference for eating healthy vegetables over those infected with any of the viruses (wouldn't you?). Hence, they gravitate in large numbers to the transgenic squash. There's more: the beetles are also now responsible for transmitting the scourge of bacterial wilt to the "healthy" transgenic plants, a disease that can be fatal to the crop. Although some farmers were initially pleased with the immunity of the genetically engineered squash to the various mosaic viruses, they began to see that nature had a grander plan: "...cucumber beetles became increasingly concentrated upon the healthy (mostly transgenic) plants, which increased exposure to and the incidence of wilt disease on the transgenic plants. This indirect cost...mitigated the overall beneficial effect..."[27]

GE summer squash and zucchini are planted in relatively limited amounts but, without labeling, you don't know what you're getting. Steer clear of conventional squash and head straight for the organic.

The List Is Somewhat Endless

According to the Non-GMO Project, an independent verifier of non-GMO products in the American marketplace, a list of other common ingredients derived from GMO risk crops are:
"Amino Acids, Aspartame, Ascorbic Acid, Sodium Ascorbate, Vitamin C, Citric Acid, Sodium Citrate, Ethanol, Flavorings

("natural" and "artificial"), Hydrolyzed Vegetable Protein, Lactic Acid, Maltodextrins, Molasses, Monosodium Glutamate, Sucrose, Textured Vegetable Protein (TVP), Xanthan Gum, Vitamins, Yeast Products."[28]

Unfortunately, genetic engineering doesn't stop at that which has already been accomplished and approved; the quest to modify our food supply is ongoing. There is much in the pipeline awaiting FDA approval.

The Arctic Apple

The old adage 'American as apple pie' is about to become tainted with...you guessed it...a GMO apple. Okanagan is a small specialty fruit company from British Columbia, Canada. Scientists there spent ten years learning how to turn off a gene in an apple so it wouldn't turn brown when it was cut open. This is *genetic manipulation* of an enzymatic process. However, enzymatic processes are *supposed* to occur in nature; they are what cause apples to turn brown, or oxidize, when they've been left out for a while...you actually *want* them to work. They are nature's way of telling you that your food is either fresh or spoiled.

When Okanagan first polled people about the Arctic apple, telling them it didn't brown or bruise, 60% said they were impressed with the product. However, when they were told it was a genetically engineered apple, 70% said they were unlikely to buy it. Disregarding the negative views of their poll group toward GMOs, the company proceeded with their product. Okanagan is now also using the technology to develop cherries, peaches and pears that don't bruise. The U.S. Apple Growers Association does *not* support this apple, but that isn't because they're specifically opposed to genetic engineering. It's because they'd like to keep the "image" of apples as "natural and healthy." This attitude may change if the apple sells well at market. The first Arctic apples varieties are going to be Golden Delicious and Granny Smith. According to Neal Carter, the president of family-run Okanagan, the genetic engineering technology "needs to be embraced if we are going to feed our planet." Really? How does that work out, exactly, when it comes to a non-browning apple?

The U.S. Agriculture Department initially registered more than 72,000 comments on the Arctic apple, most from Americans opposing its approval. The second comment period drew more than 6,100 comments, again, many of them from opponents of GMOs. Despite the negative public response, approval in the U.S. is expected this year, although the apples aren't expected to appear in supermarkets until 2015.

Okanagan has problems on their own side of the border. The British Columbia Fruit Growers Association also rejects the Arctic Apple due to the lack of independent testing and public consultation, as well as high probability of cross-pollination with non-GMO apple trees. There is also a fear of rejection of the apples by export markets. A statement by the BC Fruit Growers Association reads "(i)t seems GE crops offer more risk than benefit to mankind on all fronts."

Since we're talking apples, there's even more to be wary of. Apples top the Environmental Working Group's list of Dirty Fruits; indeed, conventional apples now rank #1 for the most pesticide residue on a fruit![29] So in addition to being genetically engineered, the Arctic apple - not being organic - will also most likely be heavily sprayed. To date, there have been no safety tests to see what effects the altered RNA of the Arctic apple might have on the human system. Who might eat these apples? *Kids?* These apples will be sliced up and pre-packaged as snack foods. "Healthy" snack foods? Keep your eyes open for this, and certainly buy organic apples.

The New Salmon On Your Dinner Plate

Scarier even than the Arctic apple is the AquaBounty genetically engineered salmon, coming soon to your dinner plate. Although we most frequently hear about GMOs in seeds and plants; it can have a presence in animals as well. Salmon is touted for its health benefits and is the most widely eaten fish in America. AquaBounty Technologies is a Massachusetts company which has been working on a genetically engineered salmon since 1996 - 18 years! They've now raised 10 generations of the fish. AquaBounty has taken the genes of an ocean eelpout - have you ever eaten that? - and inserted them into a salmon. The purpose of this genetic modification is for accelerated growth. The transgenic salmon accomplishes full growth in about half the time of a conventional salmon. The reason AquaBounty did this? To grow the fish to market size more quickly, of course. Cha-ching!

I'm guessing this new type of salmon will still look and taste like a salmon, but should it still be called 'salmon' or something else? A salmon-pout, perhaps? Should it be labeled on a menu? *Don't you want to know what you're eating?*

The AquaBounty transgenic salmon is slated to be the first genetically engineered animal that comes into the the United States food supply. The company is also developing trout and tilapia that are designed to grow faster than their conventional siblings. There are actually 35 other species of genetically engineered fish in development around the world.

In December 2012, after two years of consideration, the FDA deemed that GE salmon appeared to be safe to eat. The FDA also decided the GE salmon were unlikely to harm populations of natural salmon in the wild should they escape from the fish farms where they are raised. The reason the FDA doesn't think the salmon would do any harm in the wild is because they cannot reproduce; the GE fish are all female. (We should all pause and remember that the dinosaurs in Jurassic Park were all bred to be female too, yet somehow they managed to reproduce.)

Here's the kicker: "Research published in the Proceedings of the National Academy of Sciences found that the release of just 60 genetically engineered fish into a wild population of 60,000 could lead to the extinction of the wild population in less than 40 generations."[30] According to the National Wildlife Association, the natural lifespan of a wild salmon is 3 to 7 years. It seems a pretty hefty risk for the salmon to face extinction in a mere 120 to 280 years.[31]

Extinction of a species: that's some way to feed the planet.

Even if the FDA approves the AquaBounty salmon, consumers are approaching this media-dubbed "franken-fish" from another, more aggressive angle: urging retailers not to carry it under threat of boycott. And retailers are listening. Food chains such as Whole Foods, Trader Joe's and Target, to name a few, have committed not to carry the GE fish.

Those who observe a kosher diet may have dietary concerns with this salmon as well. Eel is not a kosher fish, but it's the source of the host DNA that is inserted into the salmon. According to the Orthodox Union, which is "the world's most recognized and trusted kosher certification," the GE salmon *is* kosher because it has fins and scales. However, there is vocal push back on this ruling, citing the Torah's prohibition on both the mixture of species as well as the eels' lack of scales. So if kashrut is a concern for you - or even if it isn't - wild salmon (or sustainably produced fish from aquaculture) might be a good option.

The overriding problem is really this: whether or not you're actually eating the transgenic fish is something you'll never know. Since GMO labeling is not mandatory in the U.S., nobody is going to tell you if you have a "franken-fish" on your plate.

The Florida Orange Crop

While Americans sip their breakfast OJ, blithely unaware, the Florida orange industry has been quietly battling *citrus greening*, an affliction that has plagued them since 2005. Going by a variety of exotic names, such as Huanglongbing or Yellow Dragon Disease, the bacteria that causes citrus greening sours oranges and makes them drop from the trees, ruining the crop. (The bacteria poses no threat to humans.)

By all media accounts the Florida orange industry resisted the idea of genetically engineering their oranges to fight the disease, mostly because they feared consumer rejection of GMOs, but genetically engineer they did. They tried a variety of measures: first modifying the oranges with DNA from a pig, then artificial DNA, then DNA from a virus, finally settling on genes from spinach. Testing has clandestinely been underway since 2010, largely funded by the orange industry itself, but the public is now going to be paying a share. In February, 2014, $125 million was appropriated from the new Farm Bill to help out with "research" for the orange growers' GMO experimentation.[32]

It's a legitimate problem: "Millions of acres of citrus crops have already been lost in the U.S. and overseas. Florida and Georgia are entirely under quarantine for citrus greening, as are portions of California, Louisiana, South Carolina and Texas. In addition, areas of the U.S. Territories of Puerto Rico and U.S. Virgin Islands are also under quarantines for citrus greening."[33]

Oranges are the most widely consumed fruit in the United States, with orange juice contributing to this statistic. There is reporting on the orange juice futures' market, and the worldwide orange market, and how the price of oranges is going to rise, all based on citrus greening. But where in the news media is there information about the genetic engineering of America's favorite fruit?

Oranges currently do not top the Environmental Working Group's "Dirty Dozen,"[34] the list that categorizes fruits and vegetables according to the amount of toxins they contain. But that could change when the EWG gets wind of the amount of pesticides that have been used in an effort to fend off this scourge of citrus greening: indeed, there's been a "tripling of pesticide applications to kill the bacteria-carrying psyllid."[35] *Triple the amount of pesticides!* The USDA has backed research for a genetically engineered solution to citrus greening,[36] and FDA regulatory approval is hoped for in 2015. Perhaps the Florida Orange Industry didn't *want* to genetically engineer their fruit, but they have gone and done it. It would have been nice if they informed their public. Here you have the heads up.

The Golden Rice Story

Perhaps the most contentiously disputed food to ever be created is genetically engineered Golden Rice. With a myriad of public health concerns on both sides of the fence, at the heart of the debate is VAD.

VAD, or Vitamin A Deficiency, is a serious health problem affecting an estimated 250 million preschool children worldwide, especially in poor countries in Africa and South-East Asia. A substantial number of pregnant women in these regions are also thought to be vitamin A deficient. The heartbreaking side effects of this deficiency are that

26

"(a)n estimated 250 000 to 500,000 vitamin A-deficient children become blind every year, half of them dying within 12 months of losing their sight."[37] According to the World Health Organization, providing Vitamin A supplementation to these areas can significantly reduce the risk of disease and death.

First, some information about vitamin A: vitamin A is a fat-soluble vitamin that is required by the human body. Fat-soluble means that dietary fat is necessary for the vitamin to be properly absorbed into the system. There are two different types of vitamin A: the first is known as preformed, and can be found in meat, poultry, fish and dairy products. The second type is provitamin A, widely known as beta-carotene, which converts to vitamin A in the body. This is found in fruits, vegetables, and other plant-based products, as well as supplements. Beta-carotene is also fat-soluble.[38]

Now, the question is: how to best supply vitamin A in order to eradicate VAD?

The World Health Organization currently has programs in place "...to combat vitamin A deficiency (that) are cheap, already available – and proven to work. They focus on methods such as educating people to grow green leafy vegetables in kitchen gardens, encouraging breastfeeding of babies, and giving supplements and fortified foods when necessary."[39] There is also UNICEF, the world's leading supplier of vitamin A supplements. "At just a few cents a capsule, Vitamin A is an extremely cost-effective, efficient method for addressing VAD. UNICEF supports 95 per cent of the world's vitamin A supplements for developing countries..."[40]

And then along came Golden Rice: unveiled in 1999, the co-architects of Golden Rice were Dr. Ingo Potrykus of the Swiss Federal Institute of Technology and Dr. Peter Beyer of the University of Freiburg in Germany. The transgenic rice was created "...(b)y inserting two genes from daffodil and one gene from a bacterium, (creating) a beta-carotene pathway into Taipei 309, a japonica rice variety."[41] Golden Rice was genetically engineered to contain beta-carotene, the precursor of vitamin A, in the DNA of each grain of rice. An unintended consequence of the genetic modification process was that the rice turned a golden color, hence the name.

Note: Rice by itself does not contain any vitamin A or beta-carotene, and only contains negligible amounts of fat which, again, are necessary for the body to absorb those vitamins.

The research, development, and evaluation processes on the bio-fortified, nutritionally-enhanced, genetically engineered Golden Rice are expected to last until 2015, making it the longest running GE food experiment.

With the knowledge they had a hot potato (no pun intended), the scientists relinquished their rights to bio-pharmaceutical company AstraZeneca, now Syngenta. There were thirty-two different companies whose technologies were used to develop, and over seventy different patents on, the rice. Six corporations, including Monsanto, Bayer and Syngenta, freely donated their technologies ostensibly to have their name on a GMO that was to do some good for humankind.[42]

Interestingly, the Golden Rice Project likens its genetic engineering technique to the same one that brought about orange carrots - selective breeding[43] - however it is quite a different thing entirely! As discussed prior in this chapter, genetic engineering is a thoroughly different process than selective breeding; one that can only take place in a lab and never in a field. (According to the World Carrot Museum, though the orange carrot is indeed a cultivated variety there is evidence that it dates back to 500 AD. Therefore, to compare its inception to genetic manipulation is clearly hogwash. [44])

So Why The Heated Debate?

Rice is a staple food in many regions of the world where VAD is a presence. So it was thought that if farmers there were to grow the Golden Rice for part of their families daily diet, then the vitamin A deficiency could be reduced, at least in some measure. However, concerns about a) the effectiveness of Golden Rice, b) the true intentions of biotech corporations in third world countries, and c) stalwart opposition to GMO's in general, continue to persist. Here are some of the arguments against moving forward with the Golden Rice project:

1 - The two basic varietals of rice are Japonica and Indica, with the first grown on dryland and the second grown in rice paddies. The current strain of Golden Rice being tested is Japonica, however it is *Indica* that is grown in regions where the vast majority of people suffer from VAD. Indeed, Japonica is known to "fare poorly in Asian fields."[45] Thus, how are the indigenous farmers to grow this rice, if indeed they can be convinced to accept it in the first place?

2 - There have been questions concerning the ability of the body to absorb the beta-carotene in Golden Rice. In an adult feeding study, servings of Golden Rice were consumed along with 10 grams of butter, which naturally contributed to high absorption of the vitamin A, and good reported results in the research.[46]   This makes sense since dietary fat is necessary to absorb beta-carotene. However, consider that the rice is to be consumed in real life settings, not in clinical situations that are supervised. Since the regions (Africa and Southeast Asia) where Golden Rice is targeted to be grown *do not* consume this type or amount of fat in their daily diet, we can presume this will not be a realistic case scenario. In addition, "dietary fat is...limited in rice-eating countries and in fact is being looked at as one possible "hidden" cause of vitamin A deficiency itself."[47]

3 - Should the absorption issues be resolved - and that is quite a hurdle - "no one knows how much beta-carotene will remain in (Golden Rice) over time when stored in normal domestic conditions. When some (Golden Rice) was sent in 2001 to scientists in Germany, they found that the level of beta-carotene was less than 1% of what it should have been. After cooking the level declined further, by 50%. This finding set back the project by many years."[48]

Beta-carotene in the form of "carotenoids are susceptible to light and oxidation. A number of studies have been conducted to determine the effects of light and air (oxygen) of harvested, stored Golden Rice. Results are highly encouraging," says the Golden Rice Project.[49] What is misleading about this research is that it was conducted in Germany, hardly the same climate as Africa or Southeast Asia, where the Golden Rice would be harvested and stored under real-life conditions. According to Dr. Michael Hansen, Senior Scientist at the Consumers Union, "...the real question is what are the beta-carotene levels in rice that has sat in storage at room temperature for month or two, similar to the local storage conditions for those who might grow this rice...no studies have been done."[50]

4 - If and when the absorption issues *and* the beta-carotene retention issues are addressed, there still exist concerns that, due to population differences (young and old, male and female, weight and age), some people will consume too much beta-carotene, and some, not enough. Beta-carotene converts to vitamin A in the body, which in extreme cases can be toxic, and "overdosing on vitamin A has been linked to an increased risk of birth defects, and in the case of smokers to an increased cancer risk."[51]

5 - Any human feeding studies that have been done on Golden Rice have been contested. Note this excerpt from a letter, signed by 32 scientists, and directed to Tufts University Medical School which organized the above feeding trials:
"We are writing to express our shock and unequivocal denunciation of the experiments being conducted...which involve the feeding of genetically modified Golden Rice to human subjects (adults and children.) We are all senior scientists / academics with a professional interest in the health and environmental effects of GMOs."[52] *The reply consisted of "The controversial Golden Rice Project has admitted on its web site that it was involved in a number of projects involving the feeding of unauthorized GM rice to both adults and children in China and the USA."*[53]

Ironically, while Golden Rice project testing escalates amidst intense debate and rancor, the issue may be less relevant as time goes by. In the Philippines, through a combined approach including vitamin A supplementation, increased efforts to fight infection, and expanded involvement by the Filipino Department of Health, "...vitamin A deficiency in young children has fallen by 25% in just 5 years – a fantastic achievement, without any GM rice;"[54] an exemplary case study.

There are also other, far less publicized crops, available that have been developed in an effort to combat the scourge of VAD. One of these is vitamin A-rich maize, a conventionally bred, hybrid corn. This orange maize is higher in beta-carotene than Golden Rice, and contains the inherent fat content needed to absorb the beta-carotene. Developed by HarvestPlus in 2010 and in limited release since 2013, this maize has quietly made its way forward. It is now being grown in Nigeria and Zambia, among other regions, with positive reviews and acceptance by the farmers. There are also varieties of vitamin A-rich cassava and vitamin A-rich sweet potatoes, both developed by methods of traditional breeding.[55]

One must question why these non-GMO crops are not more widely publicized? Could it be that without the biotech companies in the picture, the good work just goes forward quietly?

Those in opposition to Golden Rice widely feel that the "main agenda for (it) is not malnutrition but garnering greater support and acceptance for genetic engineering amongst the public, the scientific community, and funding agencies.[56] World Health Organization malnutrition expert Francesco Branca cited the lack (in 2008) of real-world studies and uncertainty about how many people will use Golden Rice, concluding "giving out supplements, fortifying existing foods with vitamin A, and teaching people to grow carrots or certain leafy vegetables are, for now, more promising ways to fight the problem."[57]

Plan B: The Genetically Engineered Banana

In June, 2014, it was suddenly announced that human trials would begin in the United States for genetically engineered, Vitamin A-enriched bananas. Developed at the Queensland University of Technology (QUT) in Australia and funded by the Bill & Melinda Gates Foundation,[58] this banana appears to be a replacement for the ill-fated Golden Rice. Following what were claimed to be successful clinical trials with Mongolian gerbils,[59] also conducted in the United States, a six week human trial at the University of Iowa was slated to begin for the purpose of testing the effects of the genetically engineered fruit on serum Vitamin A levels in humans.

With the Golden Rice fiasco losing traction, the Bill & Melinda Gates Foundation has quietly been pursuing this alternate method of genetically engineered vitamin A supplementation. It has invested close to $10 million in the project since 2005.[60]

These GE bananas should not be confused with the genetic engineering already being conducted on the varietal that is widely consumed by Americans: the "Cavendish" banana. Indeed, banana popularity is at an all time high in the United States, with per capita consumption at 10.4 pounds per year in 2010, the last available numbers published.[61] Even though there are close to 1,000 varieties of bananas in the world [62], the "Cavendish" is the one currently being cultivated for widespread export. However this is only since the late 1950's; prior to that time, Americans bought and ate only the "Gros Michel," or "Big Mike," banana. As Americans, we like our produce uniform; to us it's simply "the banana."

As the popularity of bananas surged, plantations focused on a practice known as *monocropping*. This is simply the cultivation of a single variety of crop on a farm, and is generally more labor and cost efficient for the farmer. Unfortunately, there are often bleak environmental consequences resulting from the practice. We will cover this more fully later in the book, but in the case of bananas it specifically increases susceptibility to pathogens, and with the "Big Mike" banana the move from polycropping to monocropping eventually led to a soil fungus "... colloquially known as "Panama Disease" or "fusarium wilt,"[63] that eventually wiped out the entire crop.

As a result, by 1958 the "Big Mike" needed to be replaced with another varietal, the "Cavendish," which is the type of banana we now eat. Slightly smaller and less sweet, for many of us it is the only variety of banana we know. For many decades it exhibited a greater resistance to Panama Disease. However, now the "Cavendish" as well is threatened by a new pathogen called "Tropical Race Four (TR4)," also a type of fusarium wilt. The identical mistake had been made with this banana as with the "Big Mike" - mass monocropping - and comparable dire results have come to pass. There are other ways to approach the matter, of course; "...the disease is soil-borne and the fungus can remain viable for decades and prevention includes foot baths and measures to avoid movement of infected soil and planting materials into and out of farms."[64] This, as well as a reversion to polycropping are some baseline recommendations.

The same agricultural scientist who is working on the genetically engineered, vitamin A-enriched banana for the Bill & Melinda Gates Foundation, James Dale of Queensland University, is also "working to develop new versions of the "Cavendish" that resist the fungus. He does this by inserting genetic material from other organisms into banana plants." (as succinctly explained by Mr. Gates in his blog: *"Building Better Bananas"*).[65]

However the real aim of The Gates Foundation is to develop a more *nutritious* banana.[66] An interesting question is why agricultural scientists have chosen to genetically alter the banana when one rich in the desired nutrients already exists? The "Karat" banana, which is native to Micronesia, has bright orange flesh that indicates the ultra-high levels of beta-carotene it contains (25 times more than the typical "Cavendish" banana!).[67] It can be eaten ripe, raw or steamed, as is the habit in many African countries.

No doubt the general public will be very confused when the media starts to go bananas over GMO bananas, being that there are two different types and it's difficult to keep the information straight. The vitamin A-enriched banana is a cooking banana, a plantain, and a staple food in Uganda, "where the average person consumes more than 1 kg of bananas each day."[68] Pending approval in Uganda, where it is slated to be grown by 2020, there are plans to roll out the GE banana in Rwanda, parts of the Democratic Republic of Congo, Kenya and Tanzania. Its flesh is distinctly orange-toned, a distinguishing characteristic that developers tried to diminish in an effort to bolster native acceptance. In the wave of press releases that were released to the news media in early June, 2014, there were the usual emotional entreaties of children suffering and starving in Africa and Southeast Asia due to vitamin A deficiency. And while this sad information may be verifiable, the mega-millions spent on genetically engineered bananas. unavailable to those children until 2020, if then *and* if all goes well, might be better spent in an alternative manner, and sooner. It's a lot of "ifs" and many millions that didn't pan out with the Golden Rice debacle. With this situation, as with Golden Rice, there were other options available to approach the harsh realities of vitamin deficiencies that plague the growing world population.

Vitamin A deficiency is not an isolated phenomenon, but is generally coupled with malnutrition. According to Dr. Vandana Shiva, "A far more efficient route to removing vitamin A deficiency is biodiversity conservation and propagation of naturally vitamin A rich plants in agriculture and diets."[69] While every effort must be made to obliterate malnutrition, poverty and the causes that contribute to it, the current efforts already underway by the World Health Organization and UNICEF deserve the necessary funding to continue rolling out. GMOs are not the answer.

From the food that is genetically engineered to be its own insecticide or withstand spraying of herbicides, to that which is allegedly grown to eradicate illness in the world, there's no denying that a good deal of it appears nightly on your dinner plate. This is true regardless of whether you eat at home, on the go, or dine out in the finest restaurants.

There's seemingly no end to the GMO projects on the table. There's GMO wheat, unapproved, but mysteriously appearing in American fields. Also GMO bluegrass, not a foodstuff, but recently approved and completely unregulated for planting in the U.S. There's a genetically engineered purple tomato, developed by New Energy in Canada. This is part of a new wave of GMOs that are engineered to have benefits to the consumer. "The purple tomatoes have been genetically modified to have a higher amount of anthocyanins, an antioxidant found in blueberries, blackberries and plums. It's what gives those fruit their purple colours. Anthocyanins are also said to fight cancer."[70] However, wouldn't it just make sense to eat the blueberries, blackberries and plums? There are co-factors in all of these fruits - known *and* unknown to us - that contribute to their manifold health benefits.

Consider the GMO strawberry, inserted with "anti-freeze proteins" from an Arctic winter flounder in order to improve frost resistance.[71] While the strawberry, not on the market, was reputed to have had the unintended consequence of turning electric blue, this is just a fallacy. It certainly would have been a telling way to let us know the fruit had been genetically engineered, though...if it *were* blue, would you take a bite?

With all these GMOs running rampant through the American food system it seems crazy that it is incumbent on the American people themselves, as well as grassroots movements, to decipher which foods are and are not genetically modified. Whether you believe that they are safe or not to consume, you certainly have the right to know what it is you're eating.

CHAPTER 2

WHO MAKES GMOs, AND WHY?

For time immemorial Mother Nature has held the patent rights on seeds. This of course is a facetious statement, as it is illegal in the United States to patent anything in nature. This ruling includes products of nature and/or natural DNA. However, GMOs fall into the category of *synthetic* DNA; that which is created in a laboratory and is considered new and distinct from natural DNA, and is therefore patentable. Ironically, in June, 2013, the Supreme Court decided in a landmark case that DNA that is isolated in a laboratory cannot be patented, stating "DNA is a product of nature and cannot be patented."[1] This leaves genetically modified organisms as a unique example of DNA that the United States allows patent rights on. *Confused?* Of course you are, even the government seems to be.

A Brief History Of Patents

Decades after the original Patent Act of 1790 granted protection for inventors, the 1930 Plant Patent Act was passed. With this new act Congress afforded patent protection to developers of particular new varieties of plants, for asexually reproduced plants only (this refers to ornamentals, fruit and nut trees, and other plants reproduced via budding, cutting and grafting). What is excluded are the great majority of food crops; those that reproduce with seeds.

Stay with me here.

Forty years passed by and along came the Plant Variety Protection Act of 1970. This legislation changed everything, as it not only allowed exclusive patent rights lasting for 20 - 25 years on new, distinct, uniform, and stable sexually reproduced, or tuber propagated plant varieties, but it also served as an intellectual property statute. "Intellectual property (IP) is an important legal concept which refers to creations of the mind for which exclusive rights are recognized."[2] Basic provisions of the PVP Act are that the new plant must be (1) new, (2) distinct, (3) uniform, and (4) stable. In other words, when the plant is repeatedly reproduced it will remain the same, ensuring a degree of commercial reliability. There are certain exemptions to the Act, but the one I will mention here, for we will come back to it, is that a farmer is permitted to save seed from protected varieties, and to use such saved seed in the production of a crop without infringement.[3]

In 1980, a genetic engineer by the name of Chakrabarty applied to the U.S. Patent Office and was denied a patent. He appealed and was denied again. Now his patent had nothing to do with food - it was actually for an invention dealing with oil spills - but it would prove to have broad implications for GE crops, as his discovery involved a genetically engineered bacterium. Eventually his case was overturned by a slim margin (5-4)[4] and "the Supreme Court held that a live, man-made microorganism is patentable subject matter. (This has) contributed to a revolution in biotechnology that has resulted in the issuance of thousands of patents, the formation of hundreds of new companies, and the development of thousands of bioengineered plants and food products."[5]

According to GMOAnswers.com, a website developed by the Biotech Industry to dispel "myths" surrounding GMO foods, "The United States Supreme Court confirmed in the landmark 2001 case, *J.E.M. Ag Supply v. Pioneer Hi-Bred*, that newly developed plant breeds could be patented. And the patented corn varieties at issue in that case were developed solely with simple hybridization: the mating of one corn plant with another. In short, *the patenting of biotech plant varieties does not make them different from conventionally developed varieties, it makes them the same.* (italics, mine)"[6] Huh? That's a long jump, my friends.

The world had changed, and if Mother Nature held any right to her worldwide garden, those rights now seem to be lost.

Who Makes GMOs?

With almost a quarter share of the global seed market, it's no wonder that Monsanto is the poster child for genetically modified seeds. However, they are not the only one; other U.S. companies include DuPont, Dow AgroSciences, and Land O'Lakes, while internationally there is Syngenta (Swiss), BASF (German), Group Limagrain (France), KWS AG and Bayer Crop Science (Germany) and Sakata (Japan).[7] "The top 3 companies (Monsanto, DuPont, Syngenta) together account for...47% of the worldwide proprietary seed market. ETC Group conservatively estimates that the top 3 seed companies control 65% of the proprietary maize seed market worldwide, and over half of the proprietary soybean seed market."[8]

For the most part, the biotechnology companies that produce the GE seeds also manufacture the herbicides and insecticides that are then mass-sprayed on the farmland where the crops are grown. This might seem like a conflict of interest to some, or like the perfect storm to others, mainly the stockholders of these corporations. Monsanto, for example, produces Roundup, which is the commercial name for glyphosate, the herbicide that its' genetically modified seeds are engineered to withstand. Syngenta produces Callisto, an herbicide that is applied to its GE corn seeds, as well as Reflex for glyphosate-resistant superweeds. DuPont offers a litany of products designed to help the modern farmer grow their crops - all with seeds purchased annually from DuPont, of course - with herbicides such as Enlite for soybeans and LeadOff for its corn. So this is very much a hand in glove system that works financially for the biotech seed companies, to keep the stockholders happy. And they are.

But what about the farmers? And what about the people who eat the food grown from seeds that are genetically engineered to withstand the mass-spraying of herbicides and insecticides? We'll get to those questions in a bit.

Some History On Pesticides

The widespread usage of chemicals on food crops began shortly after World War II, with the introduction of synthetic organic chemicals in the late 1940s. Ostensibly this was in an effort to save farmers from the time-consuming and backbreaking task of weeding and hence, improve their profitability. "Researchers in the early 1940s began to test (2,4-dichlorophenoxy) acetic acid (2,4-D), a new plant growth regulator chemical compound for herbicidal activity. It proved useful for selective control of broadleaf weeds without harm to grass crops such as wheat, corn and rice...By 1962, companies marketed about 100 herbicides in 6,000 different formulations (as) increased specificity for particular weed problems in individual crops under different soil and climatic conditions accounted for this rapid development of products...For most crops, the historical record shows rapid adoption of herbicides in the Untied States in the 1950s and 1960s. The adoption of herbicides was spurred by a desire to reduce weed control costs as labor became scarce and more expensive in the years after World War II."[9]

According to the National Institute of Health, "A pesticide is any substance used to kill, repel, or control certain forms of plant or animal life that are considered to be pests. Pesticides include herbicides for destroying weeds and other unwanted vegetation, insecticides for controlling a wide variety of insects, fungicides used to prevent the growth of molds and mildew...,"[10] and so on. So the widespread adoption of herbicides in the mid-20th century was well-accepted, but some insecticides had a bad rap. Consider DDT: discovered in 1939 to be extremely effective, it quickly became the most widely used insecticide in the world. A mere twenty years later, amidst serious concerns about human safety and biological effects, 86 countries banned its usage, but it took the U.S. Department of Agriculture until the 1960s to begin to regulate it, and the newly-formed Environmental Protection Agency until 1972 to ban it altogether "based on adverse environmental effects of its use, such as those to wildlife, as well as DDT's potential human health risks."[11] At this writing the there are over 350,000 pesticides registered with the EPA, and it is currently a $12.5 billion industry in the United States alone. "The current global market for pesticides (herbicides, insecticides, fungicides, nematicides and fumigants) is valued at $25.3 billion...,"[12] no small change.

How Patents, Biotech Companies and Pesticides All Come Together: GMOs

Agricultural applications account for 80% of all pesticide usage in the U.S.[13]. The Flavr Savr tomato was an example of a genetically modification for a purpose other than pesticide resistance, but there is a lengthy list of plants that are now engineered simply to resist the effects of herbicides and insecticides in the field.

The first crop to be genetically modified in the U.S. was tobacco and it remains GE until this day, with a staggering 90% of the U.S. crop a GMO. In fact, the tobacco crop takes to genetic engineering so successfully that "...(i)n biotechnology, tobacco often is used as a model plant for the testing of new procedures and in research on the function of specific genes."[14] Tobacco was also the first plant to be genetically engineered to withstand the Bt toxin.

How A Seed Is Genetically Modified

Following is a very simplified account of how a genetically modified organism is created. You can think of it as 'cutting and pasting,' just with DNA.

1- First, a desirable trait must be identified that you want your new plant (or animal) to express. This is generally resistance to herbicides (such as glyphosate) or insecticides (such as the Bt toxin), although more and more frequently subjects are being genetically engineered for growth and nutritional purposes.

2 - Once the DNA is isolated from the plant or animal with that trait (it is literally cut from cells with an enzyme), it must be combined with a vector. This is the vehicle which will allow for insertion into the host plant (or animal), and will transform it into the modified version that is desired. The vector is a circular strand of DNA (plasmid) which is usually obtained from a bacterial or viral source.

3 - The next step is to physically combine the trait DNA with the host. Using plants as our example, this is generally done by one of two methods. The most common insertion method involves a "gene gun" that uses a .22 caliber charge to shoot a metal particle coated with the trait DNA into the plant tissue. The other option is "heating...seedlings to place them under stress and make them susceptible to a bug called Agrobacterium tumefaciens. The organism specializes in invading plant DNA and tricking it into producing sugars and amino acids that feed the bacteria...Major biotech companies like Monsanto no longer (use) gene guns, switching several years ago to a targeted gene insertion process involving a strain of bacteria."[15]

4 - The process doesn't end there. "After transformation, various methods are used to differentiate between the modified plant cells

and the great majority of cells that have not incorporated the desired genes. Most often, selectable marker genes that confer antibiotic or herbicide resistance are used to favor growth of the transformed cells relative to the non-transformed cells...transformed cells are then regenerated to form whole plants using tissue culture methods."[16] Eventually, whole plants are grown expressing the desired trait.

To speed up the process of testing for traits, Monsanto has invented a high-tech machine nicknamed the "chipper" that can sliver away a piece of a genetically modified seed, and grind it up to test for the presence of the desired trait. Developed in the early 2000s, this machine is "a computer controlled seed chipper that allows seed breeders to know the exact DNA makeup of a seed before it's planted...By knowing the DNA before planting, those seeds that don't have the desired genetic makeup are never planted, but discarded...Seed chipping allows a plant breeder to list a group of characteristics he would like to see in the genetic line he is developing. Monsanto is the only seed company employing this procedure in their plant breeding program."[17] This innovation will allow Monsanto to develop genetically engineered seeds with up to 20 stacked traits in the near future. Well, golly. And I thought plants were natural.

Take note that gene insertion is not an exact science. The scientists do not always know how the genetic modification will turn out.

The two most common types of genetically engineered crops are 1) "insect-resistant" (often known as "Bt"), and 2) "herbicide-resistant." Sometimes, herbicide-resistant seeds are referred to as "Round-up Ready," in reference to the herbicide glyphosate, and its brand-name

Round-up. Monsanto was able to create its Round-up ready line by "clon(ing) a gene from a form of agrobacterium found growing at a Roundup factory. Researchers found that this particular bug's amino production was not affected by glyphosate, and they used E. coli to clone the gene responsible for this trait. Then they used a different agrobacterium — the familiar A. tumefaciens — to stick the gene into the chromosomes of plants."[18] The plants survive the spraying of glyphosate, however weeds do not.

The Bt Toxin Is A Little Bit Different

At this juncture we digress for a short primer on the Bt toxin. Bt, or Bacillus thuringiensis, is a bacterium found in soil; it is closely related to anthrax. Bt toxin is fatal against many species of insects, including moths, butterflies, flies, mosquitoes, beetles, wasps, and bees; basically insects that develop scaly wings during their adult stage. When an insect ingests the toxin, their digestive tract becomes paralyzed and it starves to death.

When a seed is genetically engineered to contain the Bt toxin, active Bt is transferred to the host seed via a vector, or vehicle, frequently also A. tumefaciens. Once the Bt toxin takes hold, it becomes synthesized into every single cell of the transgenic plant. Therefore, "the ACTIVE TOXIN IS IN EVERY PLANT CELL AND TISSUE, ALL THE TIME and cannot be washed off."[19] Then, of course, comes the spraying of the Bt insecticide, not judiciously but en-mass, as the GE crop was designed to allow. Because pests are exposed to a continuous low dosage of the Bt all around them in their environment they have a higher likelihood of developing a resistance to the toxin.

Defenders of GMOs like to point a finger at organic farmers and their usage of Bt as a natural insecticide, calling hypocrisy. However, this is another thing entirely! Bt is one of the only pesticidal options that is available to organic farmers. Because it occurs in soil naturally, Bt as a pesticide is permitted by organic standards.[20] Its use in genetic engineering and its subsequent *overuse* as a pesticide, however, has caused a profusion of woes for organic farmers. Because Bt is regarded as natural, of low toxicity and environmentally-friendly, it's been used since the 1920s and considered a good choice for organic farmers when they need to turn to a method of pest control. "The Bt bacteria, commercially available for organic farming is a preparation of weakened or most often dead bacteria, which is sprayed only in the case of high insect infestation and only onto the affected area...As far as human safety is concerned, the bacterium is only ever present on the surface of the plant and, if there were any remaining bacteria on the crop when it is prepared for consumption, it can be easily washed off."[21] The real point is that organic seeds are not genetically engineered at the cellular level to resist the spraying of the toxin. They are not tampered with at all.

In 1985, tobacco was the first crop genetically engineered to express the Bt insecticide, by the Belgian company Plant Genetic Systems (now Bayer CropScience). The tobacco was never marketed to the public.

In 1995, the EPA granted approval to grow Monsanto-produced Bt potato plants, going under the brand name NewLeaf, making them the first pesticide-producing food crop in the U.S. Horrifyingly, "some GE crops are actually classified as pesticides. For instance, the NewLeaf potato, which has since been taken off grocery shelves, was genetically engineered to produce the Bt (Bacillus thuringiensis) toxin in order to kill any pests that attempted to eat it. The actual potato was designated as a pesticide and was therefore regulated by the Environmental Protection Agency (EPA), instead of the Food & Drug Administration (FDA), which regulates food. Because of this, safety testing for these potatoes was not as rigorous as with food, since the EPA regulations had never anticipated that people would intentionally consume pesticides as food."[22]

The "NewLeaf potatoes never commanded a large share of the market, partly because several fast-food chains and chip makers declined to accept them. In the spring of 2001, Monsanto announced that NewLeaf potatoes would be discontinued so that the company could focus on more profitable products."[23] Despite the failure of the NewLeaf potato, the biotech industry was undeterred, and quickly followed up with Bt maize in 1996, and then Bt corn and Bt cotton (since 1996) and Bt soybeans. Stacked crops refer to those which are genetically engineered for both Herbicide-tolerance (HT) and Insect-resistance (Bt). According to the USDA, the use of Bt corn in the U.S. has grown from 8% in 1997 to 75% in 2013![24]

Again, Bt crops are pesticide-producing crops, expressing the Bt toxin in every cell of the plant. This is not the same as spraying an insecticide on a plant. These are not pesticides that can be washed off, but are ingested every time we eat the food. If insecticides had a bad rap in the last century, they have insidiously found their way back into every cell of our very food supply in this one.

Whether the seed is genetically engineered to produce a pesticide, or to resist the effects of herbicides that the biotech company produces and sells, or is genetically engineered to do both, this is the perfect symbiotic relationship. A product - the seed - is provided, which then requires a product you manufacture - the pesticide. It certainly was in the best corporate interest to continue on the path of creating these complementary products.

Naturally, this isn't the message a corporation would disseminate to the public in a press release or on their website. Biotech companies use phrases such as *filling needs* and *controlling problems* when describing their *partnership* with the farmers, and words like *solutions, sustainability,* and *stewardship* to describe their relationship to the land. It would seem the biotechnology companies were working hand in hand with Mother Nature herself.

GMOs As A Way To Help The Farmers

Farmers are clients of the agrichemical companies. They purchase their seeds, and then their pesticide products from them. As such, the biotech companies position themselves as being there to help the farmers in every way they can. They say they can do this with their (1) weed management, (2) pest control, and (3) yields. Is this hand in hand relationship with biotech one that is working out for the farmers?

Although biotech companies guard figures for their seed sales, suffice it to say that business is booming. But what about the farmers'?

Farming is indeed a business, and the reason GMO seed appealed to farmers in the first place was for financial and labor-efficiency concerns. All of the following come into play: seed costs, cost of farming (i.e. equipment, fertilizer, pesticides, labor, etc), crop insurance premiums, and crop value at market. Right off the bat the price of GE seed is greater; by much. For example, "While GM corn seed can cost $300 and more per bag or unit, non-GMO corn seed can cost about one-half of that."[25] In addition to price, "(t)o use patented seeds, farmers must pay a licensing fee and sign a contract with the biotechnology company that gives the farmer limited permission to plant the (GE) patented seeds for a single crop season. The licenses typically prohibit the traditional practice of saving seeds from harvested crops to plant the next season, require farmers to follow specific farming practices and sell in specific markets, and allow the seed company to inspect their fields. Preventing farmers from planting saved seeds effectively permits seed companies to artificially raise seed prices for all farmers by forcing them to buy all new seeds every year."[26] The biotech companies stringently pursue farmers who violate their licensing agreements.

So, if the cost of GE seed is higher, and a licensing agreement must be signed, where's the upside for the farmer?

Planting genetically engineered seed was supposed to make the the cost of pesticides lower, much lower, and initially they did. However over the years GMO crops have developed an increased susceptibility to the weeds and insects they were originally resistant to, resulting in what are now known as superweeds and superbugs (to be fully covered in Chapter 4). Since the resistance to pests has dissipated, farmers have actually had to increase the amount of pesticides they spray, which of course hikes up their labor demands and overall costs.

After reviewing the first 16 years of the interrelationship between GMO crops and pesticide usage in the U.S., Washington State University Professor Charles M. Benbrook found that "(o)ver the first six years of commercial use (1996-2001), HT (herbicide-tolerant) and Bt crops reduced pesticide use by 31 million pounds, or by about 2%, compared to what it likely would have been in the absence of GE crops." However, "(t)he relatively recent emergence and spread of insect populations resistant to the Bt toxins expressed in Bt corn and cotton has started to increase insecticide use, and will continue to do so..." Additionally, "(h)erbicide-tolerant crops worked extremely well in the first few years of use, but over-reliance led to shifts in weed communities and the emergence of resistant weeds that have, together, forced farmers to incrementally –
•Increase herbicide application rates (especially glyphosate),
•Spray more often, and
•Add new herbicides." [27]

Ultimately the business of farming comes down to dollars and cents; according to Modern Farmer the total cost of farming one acre of Non-GMO corn is $680.95, compared to $761.80 for GMO corn.[28] Multiply that out and the difference is big bucks for the farmer.

With increased consumer awareness of GMOs, and thus demand for non-GMO products on the rise, "interest and demand for non-GMO corn seed among US farmers is growing, according to seed suppliers who say that higher yields and returns, less cost, dissatisfaction with genetically modified traits, and better animal health are driving the demand...(and who are) selling 20 times as much conventional, non-GMO corn seed as GM this year."[29] At market, farmers can get a premium price for non-GMO crops. Additionally, there are GMO-averse markets overseas who will out-and-out reject any genetically engineered crop, giving farmers even more incentive to grow conventional crops, even if they're not organic.

And so the pendulum swings...

There are other aspects of GMO farming that seem less than reputable, but farmers who are tied to biotech seed companies have no choice. A farmer who purchases GMO seed is contractually bound in ways that would have been inconceivable to farmers of yore. Said our founding father George Washington "It is miserable for a farmer to be obliged to buy his Seeds; to exchange Seeds may, in some cases, be useful; but to buy them after the first year is disreputable."[30]

The Definition Of A Seed

Seed: "a flowering plant's unit of reproduction, capable of developing into another such plant."[31] While it's a myth that genetically modified seeds are sterile - if planted, they will grow like any other seed - what is true is that the farmers who buy them are

53

contractually forbidden from replanting them. They must purchase new seed each and every year or else they will be prosecuted under the fullest extent of the law by the biotech company that makes the seed at issue. *Don't try them*: "(a)s early as 2003, Monsanto had a department of 75 employees with a budget of $10 million for the sole purpose of pursuing farmers for patent infringement."[32]

So what has been taken as a natural right for time immemorial - replanting seed - is now a crime. The worlds' seed supply is now considered a commodity and the rights of where to grow, how to grow, or to simply save and re-grow your seed is no longer to be taken for granted...*if* you are a farmer who purchases GMO seed. Succinctly put by the Center For Food Safety "what was once a freely exchanged, renewable resource is now privatized and monopolized. Current judicial interpretations have allowed utility patents on products of nature, plants, and seeds, without exceptions for research and seed saving. This revolutionary change is contrary to centuries of traditional seed breeding based on collective community knowledge and established in the public domain and for the public good."[33]

Farmers who buy from agrichemical (aka biotech) companies are not permitted to save their seeds for replanting, a practice once fully taken for granted. They are not allowed to plant their own seed, or plant where they want to on their own property. In short, farmers lose whatever rights they have with their seeds, a travesty to say the least.

Although the figures vary it is safe to say that hundreds of farmers have been prosecuted for infringement of seed usage. On the Monsanto website it states "(s)ince 1997, we have only filed suit against farmers 145 times in the United States. This may sound like a lot, but when you consider that we sell seed to more than 250,000 American farmers a year, it's really a small number. Of these, we've proceeded through trial with only eleven farmers. All eleven cases were found in Monsanto's favor."34 Conversely, according to the Center For Food Safety "(t)o date, in the U.S., Monsanto has sued 410 farmers and 56 small farm businesses for alleged seed patent violation. Monsanto has won every single case. The company was awarded nearly $24 million from just 72 of those judgments" Additionally, "...as many as 4,500 small farmers who could not afford legal representation have been forced to accept out-of-court settlements...those farmers paid Monsanto between $85 and $160 million in out-of-court settlements."35

In addition to seed saving, agrichemical companies track if their licensed seed begins to grow where it is not authorized to be, for example, on a farm where the seed has not been purchased. Even though "seed movement" from one farm to another is acknowledged to be a normal occurrence; i.e., pollen can fly or seed can be transferred in any number of ways, via bird, animals, wind flow, water, or even human error at any stage of the crop production process, this can present a real threat to farmers who have signed GMO license agreements. Conversely, if organic or even conventional crops become tainted with GMO pollen, an entire harvest can become tainted, along with the reputation of the farmers, and their income for the season lost.

Do you recall the Plant Variety Protection Act that said farmers were going to be allowed to save their seed? Sadly, that seems to have been overruled.

Michele Jacobson

The Complicated Equation Of Farmers, GMOs and Subsidies

Some GMO crops are highly subsidized by the government. A farm subsidy is a type of payment made to a farmer or agribusiness by the federal government. Farm subsidies have been around since the 1930's, instituted by the Roosevelt administration to assist the 25% of the American population that lived and worked on family farms. (Today only 1% of the population actually lives on a farm.)

Farm subsidies do not exist to actually produce the crops. What they do is take the financial risk out of the farming system. Call them a type of insurance, or assurance, if you will. "(F)arm subsidy formulas are designed to benefit large agribusinesses rather than family farmers... Subsidy eligibility is based on the crop. More than 90 percent of all subsidies go to just five crops - wheat, cotton, corn, soybeans, and rice - while the vast majority of crops are ineligible for subsidies. Once eligibility is established, subsidies are paid per amount of the crop produced, so the largest farms automatically receive the largest checks."[36] You will note that 3 out of 5 of these crops are representative of the "big five" GMO crops grown in America today. And this is where the connection begins.

One of the problems with farm subsidies is that they encourage over-planting of certain crops, such as corn and soy. As discussed in Chapter One, derivatives of corn and soy are used in the production of highly processed foods. The United States government heavily subsidizes the GMO crops that are used to make the processed foods which, it turns out, are linked to obesity and other rampant, food-

56

related diseases (i.e. diabetes, coronary heart disease and high cholesterol)[37]. The fact that this ends up wreaking havoc on our health care system[38] turns out to be simply politics. The subsidies that are paid come directly from taxpayer dollars. Is this where you want your money to go?

Here It Is In Dollars And Cents

"Agribusiness spent $751 million over the past 5 years on lobbying congress and another $480.5 million in direct campaign contributions over the past two decades. Since 1995, taxpayers have provided $292.5 billion in direct agricultural subsidies, another $96 billion in crop insurance subsidies, and over $100 billion in subsidies to promote the growth of genetically engineered corn and soy." In fact, the bigger the farm, the larger the taxpayer subsidy, with "$32,043 (as) the average annual subsidies received by the largest 10 percent of farms between 1995 and 2012."[39] This really doesn't sound like it's helping the small family farmer.

There's More

GMO animal feed, which GMO crops is widely used for[40] is also highly subsidized, to the tune of "$84.4 billion...(from) corn subsidies (88 percent of which is now genetically modified) from 1995-2012 (and) $27.8 billion...(from) soy subsidies (94 percent of which is now genetically modified) from 1995-2012."[41]

And Still More...

"$43 million (has been) spent by the Biotechnology Industry Organization (world's largest biotech trade association) on lobbying from 2008 to 2013."[42]

GMOs As A Way To Feed The World

Staunch supporters of GMOs believe - or say they do, anyway - that genetically engineered crops are essential due to the growing world population and the need to feed it. These proponents will tell you that GMOs increase crop yields and, as such, can help to solve the problem of world hunger.

However, world hunger is largely attributable to food *accessibility*, and not the ability to grow it, therefore this argument is patently false. Besides the miseries of poverty and war which greatly influence decreased food distribution, environmental factors such as poor soil, drought and challenging climate conditions can also negatively impact crop growth.

For the most part GMOs are engineered to withstand the mass spraying of pesticides and/or to contain insecticides in their DNA. When it comes to the question of increased yields, the USDA said in its 2014 GE Crop Report that "(t)he adoption of Bt crops increases yields by mitigating yield losses from insects. However, empirical evidence regarding the effect of HT crops on yields is mixed."[43]

This best case scenario evidence was found in America and not in Africa, where GE crops specific to the sub-Saharan climate were attempted, but inferior to conventionally grown crops. GM sweet potatoes and cassava, staple foods of the African diet, were out-yielded by conventional crops and/or lost their virus resistance,[44,45,46] despite public claims to the contrary. And while Bt crops in the U.S. show confusing results - in other words, they don't so much increase yield, as protect loss from insects - the debacle of Bt cotton in third world countries is a well documented disaster, despite the public relations spin. While cotton doesn't feed the hungry, it is a cash crop and a decade after its adoption, the vast majority of those who adopted it are in debt.

Consider the case of Makhathini Flats, a region in northern South Africa. Bt cotton was introduced to the farmers there in 1998. Other than mere subsistence crops, cotton is the only cash crop grown there. With Bt cotton seeds developed by Monsanto,[47] a company called Vunisa operated as a jack-of-all-trades to the farmers: seed salesman, credit union, milling, and even marketing the cotton for them. In essence, an artificial market was created that showed high success rates to the world for the genetically engineered Bt cotton that was newly adopted by the farmers. However, "(t)he number of cotton farmers crashed once this credit dried up, dipping by more than 90% between 2001/02 and 2002/03."[48] The current situation is grim, indeed: "Yields for both irrigated and dryland farmers continue to vary widely according to fluctuating precipitation levels, hovering within 10% of what they were before Bt cotton was introduced" and "overall pest control costs remain significantly higher with Bt cotton (65% of total input costs) than with non-Bt cotton (42% of total input costs)."[49]

Furthermore, the overall debt accrued by the farmers who adopted Bt cotton was calculated at $1.2 million.[50] Once again, that's no way to feed the world.

There are conventionally bred crops already available and in the field that have been successful at increasing yields. Indeed, in studies, many non-GE bred plants have been proven to out-yield GMOs. These include crops such as maize[51], cassava[52], and beans[53] that fare well in drought conditions. These crops have been found to fare better than those that had been genetically engineered in laboratory conditions. Furthermore, the solutions that lie beyond plant genetics are preferable because they incorporate "...proven effective agroecological farm management techniques, such as building organic matter into the soil to conserve water, planting a diversity of crops, rotating crops, and choosing the right plant for the conditions."[54]

Drought Is Yet Another Challenge

Drought is not only an issue challenging the food supply worldwide, but is responsible for up to 40% of crop loss in the United States.[55] In 2011, widespread planting (deregulation) of genetically engineered drought-resistant corn was approved in the U.S. This was the first genetically engineered, *climate-adaptable* seed to be developed by Monsanto, in collaboration with BASF, a German company. The corn was genetically engineered with common soil bacteria, as well as E. coli, for both drought and antibiotic resistance. There are three strains of antibiotic resistance inherent in the seeds, although there is no clear-cut reasoning as to why this was done. However, "the USDA, in its assessment of the crop, noted that many non-GM maize varieties on the market are at least as effective as Monsanto's engineered maize variety in managing water use."[56] So, why use GE seeds at all? Good question.

Says Claire Robinson in *GMO Myths and Truths*, "Hunger is a social, political, and economic problem, which GM technology cannot address. GM is a dangerous distraction from real solutions and claims that GM can help feed the world can be viewed as exploitation of the suffering of the hungry."[57]

Still, some reputable foundations support biotechnology as the way to fight hunger in the world. The most high-profile of these may be the Bill & Melinda Gates Foundation. According to their website, the foundation supports "...research to develop more productive and nutritious varieties of the staple crops grown and consumed by farming families. These include varieties adapted to local conditions that deliver specific benefits farmers seek, such as increased yields, better nutrition, and tolerance to drought, flood, and pests." The website continues to explain how the foundation funds research for crop varieties that "better manage soil and water resources and reduce crop loss due to spoilage, weeds, pests, disease, and other threats."[58]

The Foundation strives to achieve these goals though AGRA, the Alliance for a Green Revolution in Africa, which was founded in 2006 by the Rockefeller Foundation and the Bill & Melinda Gates Foundation.[59] AGRA aims to utilize "improved agricultural technologies" (read GMOs) in order to encourage the farmers of

Africa to utilize the methods of agritechnological advances in farming via free seeds, funding, and instructional programs but there are many who are vocal about questioning these programs as a method of simply furthering the advancement of biotechnology in places where it does not belong, nor where it can really make a difference in solving the problems at hand.

One group is AGRA Watch, an off-shoot of the Seattle-based Community Alliance for Global Justice, that challenges the Bill & Melinda Gates Foundation's "questionable agricultural programs in Africa." They say "...The Gates Foundation and AGRA claim to be "pro-poor" and "pro-environment," but their approach is closely aligned with transnational corporations, such as Monsanto, and foreign policy actors like USAID. They take advantage of food and global climate crises to promote high-tech, market-based, industrial agriculture and generate profits for corporations even while degrading the environment and dis-empowering farmers. Their programs are a form of philanthrocapitalism based on biopiracy."[60] In addition, "The Gates Foundation has admittedly given at least $264.5 million in grant commitments to AGRA,[61] and also reportedly hired...a former Monsanto executive...to head up AGRA...70 percent of AGRA's grantees in Kenya work directly with Monsanto, and nearly 80 percent of the Gates Foundation funding is devoted to biotechnology.[62]

Oxfam is an international organization that works in 94 countries around the world to overcome poverty. Its stance on genetically engineered crops is that it "does not support GMOs as the solution to hunger, poverty and development."[63] In a quote that speaks volumes, Oxfam's head of advocacy and policy, Max Lawson, says "There is enough food overall in the world to feed everyone. But 900 million people still don't have enough to eat, and 1 billion people are obese. It's a crazy situation."[64] In the U.S. we have millions of acres of land where genetically engineered crops are grown for the purpose of manufacturing either nutritionally devoid, processed foods or animal feed, whereas there are entire continents that struggle with poverty and malnutrition. Many feel that it is the underlying causes of poverty, lack of education, and the lack of food accessibility that need to be addressed, rather than supplying the farmers with genetically engineered seeds. Currently, "(a)lthough GM crops are allowed to be grown in only three countries, this is likely to change in the next five years."[65]

Biofuels: Another Mitigating Factor

Biofuels are energy sources made from living things. Bioethanol - or simply 'ethanol' - is an alcohol made by fermenting the sugar and starch from plants by using yeast. The ethanol can then be utilized as fuel for vehicles in its pure form or, more frequently, mixed with gasoline to improve vehicular emissions. Corn - genetically modified, government subsidized corn - is the crop that has generally been used for this purpose.

The first corn to be genetically engineered exclusively for usage as a biofuel crop was created by Syngenta and is marketed under the brand name Enogen.[66] With a microbial gene engineered in the corns DNA, an enzyme is produced that breaks down the starch in the corn to sugar; it's like like getting a step-up on the process of making ethanol. The genetically engineered corn can increase the amount of gallons of ethanol produced in a bushel of corn by 8%.[67] Approved by the FDA in 2007[68] for both human and animal consumption - which is interesting because it isn't intended for either - it was deregulated by the USDA for planting in 2011.

Enogen corn was staunchly opposed by other corn growers as well as trade organizations that rely on corn: the Corn Refiners Association, National Grain and Feed Association, North American Millers' Association, the Pet Food Institute, and the Snack Food Association (yes, there is one!); groups that generally support the biotech industry. "The major concern of the associations is that if Enogen corn is commingled inadvertently with general commodity corn at even very low levels, it will have significant adverse impacts on food product quality and performance. Should their crops become contaminated it would have adverse effects on the quality of other foods made with corn."[69] In a public statement the North American Millers' Association expressed disappointment with the "biofuels corn," stating "...that a plant-made industrial product should have received a more thorough scientific review, adding, "Syngenta's own scientific data...shows if this corn is commingled with other corn, it will have significant adverse impacts on food product quality and performance."[70] These adverse effects include sogginess and lack of crustiness, which occur as a result from the amalayze enzyme breaking down the starch in the genetically modified Enogen corn.

Other, non-food crops are also being explored as sources for renewable energy sources. Plants have been genetically engineered with genes from marine algae to increase the levels of lipids, or oily mass, in their leaves. The algae itself is also engineered to grow more rapidly. Ecologists and environmentalists have expressed their concern about the potential for negative effects of this process on the environment, and strongly urge further studies and precaution to keep the algae from crossing over into the wild where it isn't known how it will react with other ecosystems. It is stated that "few details are publicly available because much of this information remains confidential as businesses compete to be the first to commercialize their genetically altered algae."[71] Business is business.

Back To The Problem of World Hunger

You don't have to search far to find critiques about growing crops to provide fuel when so many people are going hungry, not only in third world countries but here in America as well. While the energy crisis demands attention due, the judgement about using farmland to fuel it diverts us from what it should be used for: food production.

Again from Claire Robinson, "while parts of the world go hungry, vast tracts of cropland have been taken out of food production to grow biofuels for cars, funded by generous government subsidies. This has made food scarcer, pushing up costs. An added factor is that the growth of the biofuels industry has created a link between agriculture and fuel that never existed before."[72]

So we begin to see that GMOs aren't simply about soybeans and corn, cotton and canola at all. GMOs are a complicated equation of food scarcity versus food security, seed piracy over seed sovereignty. The simplicity of setting a seed in the soil, and growing it into the food that we can eat is no longer to be taken for granted as a natural right...although it should be, shouldn't it?

Michele Jacobson

Coming soon in
Part Two, Chapter Three:

WHY YOU WANT TO AVOID GMOs

The unequivocal question on everyone's mind is this: *are foods made from GMOs harmful to eat*? Around the world this is the cause of much contentious debate. And, depending on whom you ask, the answer may come back as a resolute *yes* or *no*.

The grim truth is that absolute *scientific research* that GMOs are harmful to the health of humans remains woefully inadequate at this time. Perhaps the burning question should really be: if further research is needed to ensure that genetically engineered foods are safe for human consumption, shouldn't it have been conducted *prior* to GMOs materializing in the vast majority of foods we find in our marketplace?

Michele Jacobson

WORKS CITED

CHAPTER ONE

1 - Leary, Warren E. "F.D.A. Approves Altered Tomato That Will Remain Fresh Longer." *nytimes.com.* The New York Times, May 19 1994. Web. Feb 2014. <http://www.nytimes.com/1994/05/19/us/fda-approves-altered-tomato-that-will-remain-fresh-longer.html>.

2 - "Cornflakes." *gmo-compass.org.* GMO Compass. 21 Nov 2007. Web. Feb 2014. <http://www.gmo-compass.org/eng/database/food/220.cornflakes.html>.

3 - "Information On GMO Sweet Corn." *nongmoproject.org.* Non-GMO Project. 2014. Web. Feb 2014. <http://www.nongmoproject.org/learn-more/sweetcorn/>.

4 -Goran MI1, Ulijaszek SJ, Ventura EE. " High fructose corn syrup and diabetes prevalence: a global perspective." Glob Public Health. 2013;8(1):55-64. doi: 10.1080/17441692.2012.736257. Epub 2012 Nov 27.

5 - "Corn." *usda.gov.* USDA Economic Research Service. 14 May 2014. Web. May 2014. <http://www.ers.usda.gov/topics/crops/corn/background.aspx#.Uu_caShNzS8>.

6 - "Is it true that most soy crops are now genetically engineered?" *whfoods.org,* the world's healthiest foods. 2001-2014. Web. Feb 2014. <http://whfoods.org/genpage.php?tname=dailytip&dbid=290>

7 - "Major Crops Grown In The United States." *epa.gov.* United States Environmental Protection Agency. 4 Apr 2013. Web. Feb 2014. <http://www.epa.gov/oecaagct/ag101/cropmajor.html>.

8 - Watrous, Monica. "On Board With Baby Food." *foodbusinessnews.net.* Food Business News. 10 Oct 2013. Web. Feb 2014. <http://www.foodbusinessnews.net/articles/news_home/Consumer_Trends/2013/10/On_board_with_baby_food.aspx?ID=%7B17F982BF-65CC-46E4-A086-B3C9598BADE5%7D&cck=1>.

9 - "FDA takes step to further reduce trans fats in processed foods." *fda.gov.* U.S. Food and Drug Administration. 7 Nov 2013. Web. Feb 2014. <http://www.fda.gov/newsevents/newsroom/pressannouncements/ucm373939.htm>.

10 - Pollack, Andrew. "In a Bean, a Boon to Biotech" *nytimes.com.* The New York Times. 15 Nov 2013. Web. Feb 2014. <http://www.nytimes.com/2013/11/16/business/in-a-bean-a-boon-to-biotech.html?pagewanted=1&_r=2&smid=tw-share&>.

11 - Seppanen, C. M., Csallany, A.S. "The effect of intermittent and continuous heating of soybean oil at frying temperature on the formation of 4-hydroxy-2-trans-nonenal and other α-, β-unsaturated hydroxyaldehydes." Journal of the American Oil Chemists' Society (2006). Volume 83, Number 2, Page 121. and "Reheating Vegetable Oil Releases Toxin." ummah.com. UMMAH. 7 May 2005. Web. Feb 2014. <http://www.ummah.com/forum/showthread.php?56026-Food-fried-In-Vegetable-Oil-May-Contain-Toxic-Compound>.

12 - "Frequently Asked Questions." sugarindustrybiotechcouncil.org. Sugar Industry Biotech Council. Web. Feb 2014. <http://www.sugarindustrybiotechcouncil.org/sugar-beet-faq>.

13 - "Sugar Beet." gmo-compass.org. GMO Compass. 22 Dec 2008. Web. Feb 2014. <http://www.gmo-compass.org/eng/grocery_shopping/crops/20.sugar_beet.html>.

14 - "Canola Facts." soyatech.com. soyatech.com. 2000-2014. Web. Feb 2014. <http://www.soyatech.com/canola_facts.htm>.

15 - ibid.

16 - Meyer, Melody. "Are You Eating GMO Cotton?" consciouslifenews.com. Conscious Life News. 5 Aug 2013. Web. Feb 2014. <http://consciouslifenews.com/eating-bt-cotton/1162301/comment-page-1/#>.

17 - "Cotton." gmocompass.org. GMO Compass. 4 Dec 2008. Web. Feb 2014. <http://www.gmo-compass.org/eng/grocery_shopping/crops/161.genetically_modified_cotton.html>.

18 - "Frequently Asked Questions About rBGH." organicvalley.coop. Organic Valley. 2014. Web. Feb 2014. <http://www.organicvalley.coop/why-organic/synthetic-hormones/about-rbgh/>.

19 - "Monsanto's Hormonal Milk Poses Serious Risks of Breast Cancer, Besides Other Cancers, Warns Professor of Environmental Medicine at the University of Illinois School of Public Health." preventcancer.com. Cancer Prevention Coalition. 21 Jun.1998. Web. Feb 2014. <http://www.preventcancer.com/press/releases/july8_98.htm>.

20 - "Hawaii Top 10 Cash Crops" norml.com. NORML and the NORML Foundation. 2014. Web. Feb 2014. <http://norml.org/legal/item/hawaii-top-10-cash-crops>.

21 - "Papaya ringspot disease." biosecurity.qld.gov.au. Biosecurity Queensland. Web. Feb 2014. <http://www.daff.qld.gov.au/__data/assets/pdf_file/0006/58857/PRSV-fact-sheet.pdf>.

22 - "Papaya Ringspot Virus-Resistant (PRVR) Papaya "Why genetically engineer virus resistance into papaya?" cornell.edu. U.S. AID. 10 Sep 2004. Web. Feb 2014. <http://absp2.cornell.edu/resources/factsheets/documents/papaya_factsheet91004.pdf>.

23 - "Papaya." hawaiiseed.org. Hawai'i Seed. Web. Feb. 2014. <http://hawaiiseed.org/local-issues/papaya/>.

24 - "Culture Of Food and Walkabouts." kumufarms.com. Kumu Farms. 2014. Web. Feb 2014. <http://kumufarms.com/information.php?info_id=10>.

25 - "2011 Hawaii Papaya Utilization and Price Down." *nass.usda.gov.* Hawaii Farm Facts. Jul. 2012. Web. Feb 2014. <http://www.nass.usda.gov/Statistics_by_State/ Hawaii/Publications/Fruits_and_Nuts/annpapFF.pdf>.

26 - Fromartz, Samuel. "Why You Should Care About Genetically Modified Alfalfa." *the atlantic.com.* The Atlantic. 1 Feb 2011. Web. Feb 2014. <http:// www.theatlantic.com/health/archive/2011/02/why-you-should-care-about-genetically-modified-alfalfa/70557/)(I>.

27 - Miruna A. Sasu, Matthew J. Ferrari, Daolin Du, James A. Winsor, and Andrew G. Stephenson. "Indirect costs of a nontarget pathogen mitigate the direct benefits of a virus-resistant transgene in wild Cucurbita." PNAS 2009. doi:10.1073/pnas.0905106106 . <http://www.pnas.org/content/early/ 2009/10/23/0905106106.full.pdf+html>.

28 - "What Is GMO?" *nongmoproject.org.* Non GMO Project. 2014. Web. Feb 2014. <http://www.nongmoproject.org/learn-more/what-is-gmo/>.

29 - "All 48 fruits and vegetables with pesticide residue data." *ewg.org.* Environmental Working Group. 2014. Web. Feb 2014. <http://www.ewg.org/ foodnews/list.php>.

30 - "Genetically Engineered Salmon: Coming Soon to a Supermarket Near You?" *oceanconservancy.org.* Ocean Conservancy. 2011. Web. Feb 2014. <http:// www.oceanconservancy.org/our-work/aquaculture/aquaculture-genetically.html>.

31 - "Chinook Salmon." *nwf.org.* National Wildlife Federation. 1996-2014. Web. Feb 2014. <http://www.nwf.org/wildlife/wildlife-library/amphibians-reptiles-and-fish/chinook-salmon.aspx>

32 - "An investment to save Florida citrus." *flcitrusmutual.com.* Florida Citrus Mutual. 2012 - 2014. Web. Feb 2014. <http://flcitrusmutual.com/news/ tbo_farmbill_061814.aspx>.

33 - Flynn, Dan. "USDA Steps Up Citrus Greening Fight As GMO Fix Looks Promising." *foodsafetynews.com.* Food Safety News. 13 Dec 2013. Web. Feb 2014. <http://www.foodsafetynews.com/2013/12/usda-steps-up-citrus-greening-fight-that-ultimately-may-require-a-gmo-fix/#.UvV0kSj6TS8>.

34 - *ibid,* 29.

35 - Harmon, Amy. "A Race to Save the Orange by Altering Its DNA." *nytimes. com.* The New York Times. 27 Jul 2013. Web. Feb 2014. <http://www.nytimes.com/ 2013/07/28/science/a-race-to-save-the-orange-by-altering-its-dna.html?_r=0>.

36 - Flynn, Dan. "USDA Steps Up Citrus Greening Fight As GMO Fix Looks Promising." *merid.org.* Meridian Institute. 16 Dec 2013. Web. Feb 2014. <http:// www.merid.org/en/Content/News_Services/Food_Security_and_AgBiotech_News/ Articles/2013/Dec/16/HLB.aspx>.

37 - "Micronutrient deficiencies." *who.int.* World Health Organization. 2014. Web. Feb 2014. <http://www.who.int/nutrition/topics/vad/en/>.

38 - "Vitamin A: Fact Sheet for Consumers." *nih.gov.* National Institutes of Health. 5 Jun 2013. Web. Feb 2014. <http://ods.od.nih.gov/factsheets/VitaminA-QuickFacts/>.

39 - "Golden Rice: Scientific Realities." *gmwatch.org.* GM Watch. 13 Jan 2014. Web. Feb 2014. <-http://www.gmwatch.org/index.php/news/archive/2014/15255-golden-rice-scientific-realities>.

40 - Dwivedi, Archana. "Eliminating Vitamin A Deficiency." *unicef.org.* Unicef. Web. Feb 2014. <http://www.unicef.org/nutrition/23963_vitaminadeficiency.html>.

41 - "Grains of delusion: Golden rice seen from the ground." *grain.org.* Grain. 25 Feb 2001. Web. Feb 2014. <http://www.grain.org/article/entries/10-grains-of-delusion-golden-rice-seen-from-the-ground>.

42 - *ibid.*

43 - "How does Golden Rice work?" *goldenrice.org.* Golden Rice Project. 2005-14. Web. Feb 2014. <http://www.goldenrice.org/Content2-How/how.php>.

44 - "History of the Carrot: The Road to Domestication... AND the Colour Orange!" carrotmuseum.co. World Carrot Museum. Web. Feb 2014. <http://www.carrotmuseum.co.uk/history5.html#orange>.

45 - Enserink, Martin. "Tough Lessons From Golden Rice." *fbae.org.* Foundation for Biotechnology Awareness and Education. 2008. Web. Feb 2014. <http://fbae.org/2009/FBAE/website/news_tough-lessons-from-golden-rice.html>.

46 - Hansen, Michael, Ph.D. "Golden Rice Myths." *gmwatch.org.* GM Watch. 28 Aug 2013. Web. Feb 2014.<http://www.gmwatch.org/index.php/news/archive/2013/15023-golden-rice-myths>.

47 - *ibid,* 41.

48 - *ibid,* 39.

49 - "Testing the performance of Golden Rice." *goldenrice.org.* Golden Rice Project. 2005-14. Web. Feb 2014. <http://www.goldenrice.org/Content2-How/how8_tests.php>

50 - *ibid,* 46.

51 - "Vitamin A: Fact Sheet for Health Professionals." *nih.gov.* National Institutes of Health. 5 Jun 2013. Web. Feb 2014. <http://ods.od.nih.gov/factsheets/VitaminA-HealthProfessional/>.

52 - "Scientists Protest Unethical Clinical Trials of GM Golden Rice." *i-sis.org.* Institute of Science in Society. 16 Feb 2009. Web. Feb 2014 <http://www.i-sis.org.uk/SPUCTGM.php>.

53 - "Golden Rice Humanitarian Board admits to human feeding trials." *gmfreecymru.org.* GM-Free Cymru. 14 Mar. 2009. Web. Feb 2014. <http://www.gmfreecymru.org/news/Press_Notice14mar2009.htm>.

54 - "7th National Nutrition Survey: 2008 Biochemical Survey Component." *fnri.dost.gov.* Food and Nutrition Research Institute. 2008. Web. Feb. 2014. <http://www.fnri.dost.gov.ph/images/stories/7thNNS/biochemical/biochemical_vad.pdf>.

55 - "Vitamin A Maize." *harvestplus.org.* Harvest Plus. 2004-2009. Web. Feb 2014. <http://www.harvestplus.org/content/vitamin-maize>.

56 - *ibid,* 41.

57 - "Golden Rice "could save a million kids a year." *gmwatch.org.* GM Watch. May 2012. Web. Feb 2014. <http://www.gmwatch.org/index.php/golden-rice-could-save-a-million-kids-a-year>.

58 - "GMO bananas enriched with vitamin A to benefit millions in Africa set for human trials in US." *geneticliteracyproject.org.* Genetic Literacy Project. 17 Jun 2014. Web. Jun 2014. <http://www.geneticliteracyproject.org/2014/06/17/gmo-

bananas-enriched-with-vitamin-a-to-benefit-millions-in-africa-set-for-human-trials-in-us/>.

59 - "Super bananas – world first human trial." *www.qut.edu*. Institute for Future Environments. 16 Jun 2014. Web. Jun 2014. <https://www.qut.edu.au/institute-for-future-environments/about/news-events/news?news-id=74077>.

60 - *ibid.*

61 -"Bananas and apples remain America's favorite fresh fruits." *ers.usda.gov*. United States Department of Agriculture Economic Research Service. 27 Aug 2012. Web. Jun2014. <http://www.ers.usda.gov/data-products/chart-gallery/detail.aspx?chartId=30486#.U7REsyj6TS8>.

62 - "All About Bananas." *bananalink.org*. BananaLink. Web. Jun 2014. <http://www.bananalink.org.uk/all-about-bananas>.

63 - "The History of the Banana: Is the End Nigh?" *cwh.ucsc.edu*. History of the Banana: 1800 to Present. Web. Jun 2014. <http://cwh.ucsc.edu/bananas/Site/Modern%20History%20of%20the%20Banana.html>.

64 - Thuburn, D. "Disease threatens world's bananas, says UN." *phys.org*. PHYS.ORG. 14 Apr 2014. Web. Jun2014. < http://phys.org/news/2014-04-disease-threatens-world-bananas.html#jCp>.

65 - Gates, Bill. "A Bunch Of Reasons: Building Better Bananas." *gatesnotes.com*. gatesnotes: The Blog Of Bill Gates. 30 Jan 2012. Web. Jun2014. <http://www.gatesnotes.com/Development/Building-Better-Bananas>.

66 - *ibid.*

67 - "Karat Gold - the life-saving banana of Pohnpei." *new-ag.info*. New Agriculturalist. May 2008. Web. Jun 2014. <http://www.new-ag.info/en/focus/focusItem.php?a=427>.

68 - Dale, J. "Optimisation of Bioavailable Nutrients in Transgenic Bananas." *grandchallenges.org*. Grand Challenges In Global Health. 2003-2013. Web. Jun 2014. <http://www.grandchallenges.org/ImproveNutrition/Challenges/NutrientRichPlants/Pages/Bananas.aspx>.

69 - Shiva, Vandana. " The "Golden Rice Hoax" - When Public Relations replaces Science." (undated letter, 2001.) Web. Feb 2014. <http://online.sfsu.edu/rone/GEessays/goldenricehoax.html>.

70 - "Cancer fighting purple tomatoes harvested in Leamington." *cbc.ca*. CBC News. 28 Jan 2014. Web. Feb 2014. <http://www.cbc.ca/news/canada/windsor/cancer-fighting-purple-tomatoes-harvested-in-leamington-1.2514078>.

71 - Firsov, A.P., and Dolgov, S.V. "Agrobacterial Transformation and Transfer of the Antifreeze Protein Gene of Winter Flounde to the Strawberry." *Proc. of the Eucarpia Sypm. on Fruit and Breeding Genetics*: (1999). pp 581-6. Web. <http://www.salmone.org/wp-content/uploads/2011/12/fragola-pesce.pdf>.

CHAPTER TWO

1 - "Association for Molecular Pathology et al v. Myriad Genetics Inc., et al." *supremecourt.gov*. Supreme Court of the United States. Oct. 2012. Web. Feb. 2014.<http://www.supremecourt.gov/opinions/12pdf/12-398_1b7d.pdf>.

2 - Raysman, R. Pisacreta, E. Ostrow, S., Adler, K. *Intellectual Property Licensing: Forms and Analysis*. Law Journal Press, 2014. Web.

3 - "What is the U.S. Plant Variety Protection Act (PVPA)?" *datcp.wi.gov*. Wisconsin Department of Agriculture, Trade and Consumer Protection. Jan 2012. Web. Feb 2014. <http://datcp.wi.gov/uploads/Plants/pdf/BrownBagSeed.pdf>.

4 - "Diamond v. Chakrabarty - 447 U.S. 303 (1980)." *supreme.justia.com*. Justia U.S. Supreme Court. Web. Feb 2014. <http://supreme.justia.com/cases/federal/us/447/303/case.html>.

5 - Robinson, D. and Medlock, N. *"Diamond v. Chakrabarty: A Retrospective on 25 Years of Biotech Patents."* Intellectual Property & Technology Law Journal, Volume 17, Number 10: Oct 2005 <http://www.bannerwitcoff.com/_docs/library/articles/Chakrabarty.pdf>.

6 - "Ask Us Anything About GMOs!" *gmoanswers.com* GMO Answers. Dec 2013. Web. Feb 2014. <http://gmoanswers.com/ask/you-claim-gmo-foods-are-essentially-same-non-gmo-and-therefore-safe-without-proof-other-hand>.

7 - "The world's top 10 seed companies: who owns Nature?" *gmwatch.org*. GMWatch. Web. Feb 2014.<http://www.gmwatch.org/gm-firms/10558-the-worlds-top-ten-seed-companies-who-owns-nature>.

8 - *ibid.*

9 - Gianessi, L. and Reigner, N. "The Value of herbicides in U.S. Crop Production." *Weed Technology* 21: 559-566. 2007. <http://croplifefoundation.files.wordpress.com/2012/05/weed-technology-article-2007.pdf>.

10 - "Pesticides." *niehs.com*. National Institute of Environmental Health Services. 24 Jun 2013. Web. Feb 2014. <http://www.niehs.nih.gov/health/topics/agents/pesticides/>.

11 - "DDT - A Brief History and Status." *epa.gov*. U.S. Environmental Protection Agency/Pesticides: Topical and Chemical Fact Sheets. 2014. Web. Feb 2014. <http://www.epa.gov/pesticides/factsheets/chemicals/ddt-brief-history-status.htm>.

12 - Ibrahim, M., Griko, N., Junker, M., and Bulla, L. "Bacillus thuringiensis." *Bioeng Bugs*. Jan-Feb; 1(1): 31-50. 2010. <http://www.ncbi.nlm.nih.gov/pmc/articles/PMC3035146/>.

13 - "Pesticides Industry Sales and Usage: 2006 and 2007 Market Estimates." *epa.gov*. United States Environmental Protection Agency. 2011. Web. Feb 2014. <http://www.epa.gov/opp00001/pestsales/07pestsales/market_estimates2007.pdf>.

14 - "Tobacco." *gmo-compass.org*. GMO Compass. 29 Jul 2010. Web. Feb 2014. <http://www.gmo-compass.org/eng/database/plants/304.tobacco.html>.

15 - Boyle, R. "How To Genetically Modify A Seed, Step By Step." *popsci.com.* Popular Science. 24 Jan 2011. Web. Feb 2014. <http://www.popsci.com/technology/gallery/2011-01/gallery-how-make-genetically-modified-seed/?image=4>.

16 - "Process of Developing Genetically Modified (GM) Crops." *nepadbiosafety.net.* ABNE: African Biosafety Network of Expertise. 2010. Web. Feb 2014. <http://www.nepadbiosafety.net/subjects/biotechnology/process-of-developing-genetically-modified-gm-crops>.

17 - Hildebrant, Dan. "Seed chipper speeds up genetic progress for many crops." *farmandranchguide.com.* Farm & Ranch Guide. 26 Sep 2012. Web. Feb 2014. <http://www.farmandranchguide.com/news/agri-tech/seed-chipper-speeds-up-genetic-progress-for-many-crops/article_74848bbc-080a-11e2-9880-0019bb2963f4.html>.

18 - *ibid,* 15.

19 - "Bt in organic farming and GM crops - the difference." *gmwatch.* GM Watch. Web. Feb 2014. <http://www.gmwatch.org/latest-listing/40-2001/1058-bt-in-organic-farming-and-gm-crops-the-difference->.

20 - "Organic Farmers Threatened by GE Crops." *organicconsumers.org.* Organic Consumers Association. Web. Feb 2014. <http://organicconsumers.org/Organic/ov3.cfm>.

21 - *ibid,* 19.

22 - "Genetic Engineering." *sustainabletable.org.* Grace Communications Foundation. 2014. Web. Feb 2014. <http://www.sustainabletable.org/264/genetic-engineering>.

23 - "Discontinued Transgenic Crops." *cls.casa.colostate.edu.* Transgenic Crops: An Introduction and Resource Guide. 11 Mar 2004. Web. Feb 2014. <http://cls.casa.colostate.edu/transgeniccrops/defunct.html>.

24 - "Adoption of Genetically Engineered Crops in the U.S." *ers.usda.gov.* United States Department of Agriculture Economic Research Service. 9 Jul 2013. Web. Feb 2014. <http://www.ers.usda.gov/data-products/adoption-of-genetically-engineered-crops-in-the-us/recent-trends-in-ge-adoption.aspx#.UyJkKCj6TS9>.

25 - Roseboro, K. "Demand growing for non-GMO corn seed." *non-gmoreport.com.* The Organic & Non-GMO Report. 4 Jan 2013. Web. Feb 2014. <http://www.non-gmoreport.com/articles/january2013/Demand-growing-for-non-GMO-corn-seed.php#sthash.1YYFCVVK.dpuf>.

26 - "Consolidation and Intellectual Property Rights in the Seed Industry." *foodandwaterwatch.org.* Food and Water Watch. Mar 2011. Web. Feb 2014. <http://documents.foodandwaterwatch.org/doc/Antitrust-Seeds-web.pdf>.

27 - Clark, B. "Summary of Major Findings and Definitions of Important Terms "Impacts of genetically engineered crops on pesticide use in the U.S. – the first sixteen years" by Charles M. Benbrook." *news.cahnrs.wsu.edu.* Washington State University: College of Agricultural, Human, and Natural Resource Sciences. 1 Oct 2012. Web. Feb 2014. <http://news.cahnrs.wsu.edu/2012/10/01/summary-of-major-findings-and-definitions-of-important-terms/>.

28 - Royte, E. "The Post-GMO Economy." *modernfarmer.com*. Modern Farmer. 6 Dec 2013. Web. Feb 2014. <http://modernfarmer.com/2013/12/post-gmo-economy/>.

29 - *ibid*, 25.

30 - George Washington,"Letter to farm manager William Pearce" (November 16, 1794).

31 - "seed." *oxforddictionaries.com*. Oxford Dictionaries. 2014. Web. Feb 2014. <http://www.oxforddictionaries.com/us/definition/american_english/seed>.

32 - "Seed Giants vs. U.S. Farmers." *centerforfoodsafety.org*. Center For Food Safety. 2013. Web. Feb 2014. <http://www.centerforfoodsafety.org/files/seed-giants_final_04424.pdf>.

33 - *ibid.*

34 - "Saved Seed and Farmer Lawsuits." *monsanto.com*. Monsanto. 2002-2014. Web. Feb 2014. <http://www.monsanto.com/newsviews/pages/saved-seed-farmer-lawsuits.aspx>.

35 - Lo, P. "Monsanto Bullies Small Farmers Over Planting Harvested GMO Seeds." *corpwatch.org*. Corp Watch. 24 Mar 2013. Web. Feb 2014. <http://www.corpwatch.org/article.php?id=15825>.

36 - Reidl, B.M. "How Farm Subsidies Harm Taxpayers, Consumers, and Farmers, Too." *heritage.org*. The Heritage Foundation. 20 Jun 2007. Web. Feb 2014. <http://www.heritage.org/research/reports/2007/06/how-farm-subsidies-harm-taxpayers-consumers-and-farmers-too>.

37 - Willett WC, Koplan JP, Nugent R, et al. Prevention of Chronic Disease by Means of Diet and Lifestyle Changes. In: Jamison DT, Breman JG, Measham AR, et al., editors. Disease Control Priorities in Developing Countries. 2nd edition. Washington (DC): World Bank; 2006. Chapter 44. <http://www.ncbi.nlm.nih.gov/books/NBK11795/>.

38 - "Rising Health Care Costs are Unsustainable." *cdc.gov*. Workplace Health Promotion. 23 Oct 2013. Web. Feb 2014. <http://www.cdc.gov/workplacehealthpromotion/businesscase/reasons/rising.html>.

39 - "Factory Farms: Taxpayers Pay, Politicians Take, Agribusiness Profits." *organicconsumers.org*. Organic Consumers Association. 9 Oct 2013. Web. Feb 2014. <(http://www.organicconsumers.org/articles/article_28489.cfm>.

40 - Beville, R. "How Pervasive are GMOs in Animal Feed?" *gmoinside.org*. GMO Inside. 16 Jul 2013. Web. Feb 2014. <http://gmoinside.org/gmos-in-animal-feed/>.

41 - *ibid*, 39.

42 - *ibid*, 39.

43 - Fernandez-Cornejo, J., Wechsler, S.J., Livingston, M. and Mitchell, L. "Genetically Engineered Crops in the United States." *Economic Research Report* No. (ERR-162) 60 pp, Feb 2014. Web.

44 -Gathura G. "GM technology fails local potatoes." *mindfully.org*. The Daily Nation (Kenya). 29 Jan 2004. <http://bit.ly/KPQPxL>.

45 - " Monsanto failure." *newscientist.com*. New Scientist. 7 Feb 2004. <http://www.newscientist.com/article/mg18124330.700-monsanto-failure.html>.

46 - "Danforth Center cassava viral resistance update." *danforthcenter.org*. Donald Danforth Plant Science Center. 30 Jun 2006. Web. Feb 2014. <http://www.danforthcenter.org/news-media/Danforth-Center-Cassava-Viral-Resistance-Review-Update>.

47 - "Cotton Seeds." *monsanto.com*. Monsanto. 2002-2014. Web. Feb 2014. <http://www.monsanto.com/products/pages/cotton-seeds.aspx>.

48 - Fok, M., Hofs, J.L., Gouse, M., Kirsten, J. "Contextual appraisal of GM cotton diffusion in South Africa." Life Science International Journal, Vol. 1, No. 4 (2007): Page 468-482 CIRAD, France.

49 -Schnurr, M. "Inventing Makhathini: Creating a prototype for the dissemination of Genetically Modified crops into Africa." Geoforum (Impact Factor: 1.93). 06/2012; 43(4):784–792. DOI:10.1016/j.geoforum.2012.01.005. <http://matthewschnurr.com/wp-content/uploads/2012/08/Geoforum.pdf>.

50 - deGrassi A. "Genetically Modified Crops and Sustainable Poverty Alleviation in Sub-Saharan Africa: An Assessment of Current Evidence." *biosafety-info.net*. Jun 2003. Web. Feb 2014. <http://www.biosafety-info.net/file_dir/1919248844e4526271.pdf>.

51 - Gillam C. "DuPont says new corn seed yields better in droughts." *reuters.com*. Reuters. 5 Jan 2011. Web. Feb 2014. <http://reut.rs/Li0c5B>.

52 - "Farmers get better yields from new drought-tolerant cassava." *old.iita.org*. International Institute of Tropical Agriculture (IITA). 3 Nov 2008. Web. Feb 2014. <http://bit.ly/L3s946>.

53 - Yao S. "ARS releases heat-tolerant beans." *ars.usda.gov*. USDA Agricultural Research Service. 30 Jun 2010. Web. Feb 2014. <www.ars.usda.gov/is/pr/2010/100630.htm>. and Berthelsen, J. "A New Rice Revolution on the Way?" *asiasentinel.com*. asia sentinel. 17 Jan 2011. Web. Feb 2014. <http://www.asiasentinel.com/econ-business/a-new-rice-revolution-on-the-way/>.

54 - Fagan, J., Antoniou, M., Robinson, C. "GMO Myths and Truths, 2nd Edition." *earthopensource.org*. Earth Open Source. 2014. Web. Feb 2014. <http://earthopensource.org/files/pdfs/GMO_Myths_and_Truths/GMO_Myths_and_Truths_1.3b.pdf>.

55 - "U.S. Drought 2012: Farm and Food Impacts." *ers.usda.gov*. United States Department of Agriculture Economic Research Service. 26 Jul 2013. Web. Feb 2014. <http://www.ers.usda.gov/topics/in-the-news/us-drought-2012-farm-and-food-impacts.aspx#.Uz1wOjj6TS8>.

56 - *ibid*, 54.

57 - *ibid*, 54.

58 - "What We Do: Agricultural Development Strategy Overview." *gatesfoundation.org*. Bill & Melinda Gates Foundation. 1999-2014. Web. Feb 2014. <http://www.gatesfoundation.org/What-We-Do/Global-Development/Agricultural-Development>.

59 - "Our Story." *agra.org*. AGRA: Growing Africa's Agriculture. 2014. Web. Feb 2014. <http://www.agra.org/who-we-are/#.U6sWlyj6TS8>.

60 - "AGRA Watch" *seattleglobaljustice.org.* Community Alliance for Global Justice. 2008-2014. Web. Feb 2014. <http://www.seattleglobaljustice.org/agra-watch/>.

61 - "Fact Sheet." *gatesfoundation.org.* Bill & Melinda Gates Foundation. 2010. Web. Feb 2014. <www.gatesfoundation.org/about/Documents/BMGFFactSheet.pdf>.

62 - "Global Small Farmers Denounce Gates Foundation Purchase of 500,000 Monsanto Stock Shares." *organicconsumers.org.* Organic Consumers Association. 13 Sep 2010. Web. Feb 2014. <http://www.organicconsumers.org/articles/article_21606.cfm>.

63 - "Oxfam International's position on transgenic crops." *oxfam.org.* Oxfam International. 2014. Web. Feb 2014. <http://www.oxfam.org/en/grow/category/freetags/gmos#sthash.eMeBjRsr.dpuf>.

64 - Doucleff, M. "Where In The World Is The Best Place For Healthy Eating?" *npr.org.* NPR: The Salt. 15 Jan 2014. Web. Feb 2014. <http://www.npr.org/blogs/thesalt/2014/01/14/262465619/where-in-the-world-is-the-best-place-for-healthy-eating>.

65 - Tran, M. "Vandana Shiva: 'Seeds must be in the hands of farmers'." *theguardian.com.* Global Development. 25 Feb 2013. Web. Feb 2014. <http://www.theguardian.com/global-development/2013/feb/25/vandana-shiva-seeds-farmers>.

66 - "Enogen." *syngenta.com.* Syngenta. 2012. Web. Feb 2014. <http://www.syngenta.com/country/us/en/agriculture/seeds/corn/enogen/Pages/enogen-home.aspx>.

67 - "Enogen In Action." *bluetoad.com.* Seed Today - 3Q_11.2011. Web. Feb 2014. <http://www.bluetoad.com/display_article.php?id=823561>.

68 - "EnogenTM Corn Technology Q&A." *redbarnenterprises.com.* Enogen. May 2011. Web. Feb 2014. <http://www.redbarnenterprises.com/images/Agronomy%20Info/Corn/Enogen%20Grower%20QA%20FINAL%205_27_2011_1.pdf>.

69 - "USDA Fully Deregulates GE 'Ethanol Corn'." *foodsafetynews.com.* Food Safety News. 12 Feb 2011. Web. Feb 2014. <http://www.foodsafetynews.com/2011/02/usda-fully-deregulates-ethanol-corn/>.

70 - "Grain millers disappointed with deregulation of "biofuels corn"." *agranet.com.* Food Chemical News. 14 Feb 2011. Web. Feb 2014. <http://www.agranet.com/portal2/fcn/home.jsp?template=newsarticle&artid=20017849037&pubid=ag096>.

71 - Caldwell, E. "Ecologist: Genetically Engineered Algae For Biofuel Pose Potential Risks That Should Be Studied." *researchnews.osu.edu.* The Ohio State University Research and Innovation Communications. 2012. Web. Feb 2014. <http://researchnews.osu.edu/archive/GEalgae.htm>.

72 - *ibid,* 54.

ABOUT THE AUTHOR

Michele Jacobson is a Certified Clinical Nutritionist and food writer. A member of the NOFA - New Jersey Public Policy and Advocacy Committee, she supports mandatory labeling and has been researching, writing about and speaking on the topic of GMOs for over three years.

Her first book, *Just Because You're An American Doesn't Mean You Have To Eat Like One!*, examines the ill effects of the Western Diet on the health of Americans, as well as the role the media has played in sensationalizing and misinforming the public about food. It also explores the health benefits of traditional diets of the world.

GMOs: What's Hidden In Our Food is her second book. It will be published as a 3 part series due to the evolving landscape of the topic.

Please visit her website and blogs at
www.nutritionprescription.biz

Cover design by Debbi Wraga

Author photograph by Amy Sinicin

www.ingramcontent.com/pod-product-compliance
Lightning Source LLC
Chambersburg PA
CBHW060516280326
41933CB00014B/2985